Foundation Themes

Senses

Barbara J Leach

Text © 2003 Barbara J Leach
© 2003 Scholastic Ltd

Designed using Adobe InDesign

Published by Scholastic Ltd
Villiers House
Clarendon Avenue
Leamington Spa
Warwickshire CV32 5PR

Visit our website at www.scholastic.co.uk

Printed by Belmont Press

1 2 3 4 5 6 7 8 9 0   3 4 5 6 7 8 9 0 1 2

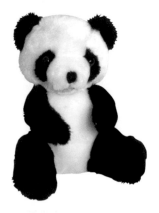

Author
Barbara J Leach

Editor
Victoria Lee

Assistant Editor
Saveria Mezzana

Series Designer
Joy Monkhouse

Designer
Erik Ivens

Illustrations
Andy Robb/Beehive Illustration

Cover photography
© Ray Moller/Scallywags

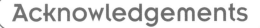

Acknowledgements

The publishers gratefully acknowledge permission to reproduce the
following copyright material:

Qualifications and Curriculum Authority for the use of extracts from the
QCA/DfEE document *Curriculum Guidance for the Foundation Stage*
© 2000 Qualifications and Curriculum Authority

Every effort has been made to trace copyright holders and the publishers
apologise for any inadvertent omissions.

British Library Cataloguing-in-Publication Data A catalogue record for
this book is available from the British Library.

ISBN 0 439 98463 7

Contents

Chapter 1

Sight

Chapter 2

Touch

Chapter 3

Hearing

Chapter 4

Taste

Foundation Themes

Senses

Contents

Chapter 5

Smell

Circle time

Displays

Photocopiables

Rhymes

Songs

Activities

Introduction

This book forms part of a series covering a wide range of popular early years themes, including 'Seasons', 'Ourselves', 'The seaside', 'Colours', 'Senses' and many more. Each book will provide practical activities to support the Early Learning Goals identified by the Qualifications and Curriculum Authority (QCA) and the Stepping Stones leading to these Goals.

The *Foundation Themes* series is designed to be used by all those working with three- to five-year-old children – including childminders, playgroup leaders, nursery nurses, and nursery and Reception teachers – in a range of settings and situations. Each book will provide cross-curricular guidance within its specific theme to support a comprehensive and successful delivery of the Foundation Stage curriculum through that theme. The books will offer advice and guidance on all aspects of curriculum delivery, from planning for equal opportunities (including special educational needs, ethnic and cultural diversity, and gender), to assessment (both formal and informal), and will include ideas for interactive displays to further the children's learning.

The activities themselves are aimed at four-year-olds, with suggestions for both offering support to younger children, so that they are able to take full advantage of the learning opportunities presented, and extending the ideas to further challenge older children. Also included are some separate activities, suitable for whole-group circle time, along with a selection of photocopiable resource sheets to provide a range of new poems and songs, templates and activity sheets.

Using a theme

The Foundation Stage curriculum is divided into six Areas of Learning, which together form a comprehensive and integrated guidance for early years practitioners. Presenting this curriculum through a theme gives the child, the parents or carers and the practitioner a focus for their attention. Activities can be planned, resources gathered and special arrangements made for inviting in visitors, taking special trips or holding special events, to provide a lively and interesting programme of learning across all areas of the curriculum. Sometimes a topic will be planned to suit a particular event in the year, and sometimes it might be initiated by the interests of a particular child or group of children. Often it will be part of a series of topics that you will have chosen to capture the children's interest and imagination, while helping them to make progress towards, and sometimes beyond, the Early Learning Goals.

Some topics may be short term and last for only a week or so, others might be planned to last up to a month or more. Either way, it is important to maintain the children's motivation to learn, by constantly providing fresh ideas to stimulate and encourage their learning. This is what this series is designed to help you with, each book providing 60 different activities, with further starting-points for related activity ideas.

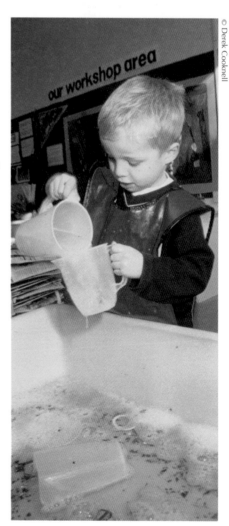
© Derek Cooknell

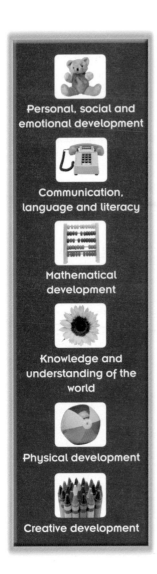

Personal, social and emotional development

Communication, language and literacy

Mathematical development

Knowledge and understanding of the world

Physical development

Creative development

How to use this book

This book is divided into five activity chapters, each referring to one sense: 'Sight', 'Touch', 'Hearing', 'Taste' and 'Smell'. Each chapter contains 12 main activities, covering all Areas of Learning in equal measure. Thus, there are two activities relating to aspects of Personal, social and emotional development, two to Communication, language and literacy, two to Mathematical development, and so on across the whole curriculum.

The activities cover a variety of Early Learning Goals within each Area of Learning (see logos in the left-hand panel) and provide for progression through various Stepping Stones within each chapter. This means that the early Stepping Stones will be covered within the first few activities in each chapter, and the later ones towards the ends of the chapters. Each Stepping Stone is colour-coded to show whether the activity is at the simplest level (yellow), at a higher level (blue) or at the highest level (green), to match the colours used to show progression in the document *Curriculum Guidance for the Foundation Stage* (QCA).

Each activity can be used as a stand-alone idea or as part of a planned sequence within the theme of 'Senses'. Some of the activities are supported by photocopiable resource sheets, which you can find on pages 89–96.

The photocopiable sheets

The photocopiable sheets are each referred to within the activity to which they are appropriate, though they may also be used independently if desired as they are largely self-explanatory (any necessary instructions for their use are given in the relevant activity). They include six new rhymes and songs – one of each on the general theme of 'Senses', and a further one of each dealing specifically with each of the five senses. For ease of delivery, the songs are all set to well-known tunes, such as 'Lavender's Blue' and 'Frère Jacques'. You could consider introducing your 'Senses' theme by singing the song 'Things I can do' on the photocopiable sheet on page 86 and sharing the rhyme 'Wouldn't it be a funny world?' on the photocopiable sheet on page 83.

Links with home

It is vital that practitioners and parents or carers work together during the children's early years, in order to ensure a smooth transition from home to setting. Suggestions are made at the end of each activity, under 'Home partnership' on ways to maintain the necessary effective communication, so that the children's learning and development may be supported and developed both within the setting and at home.

Health and safety

While it is important that children use all their senses in their learning, it is essential that you ensure the safety of all the children in your care. Therefore, you must carry out a thorough check for any allergies, dietary requirements or medical conditions before undertaking any activity that involves tasting, smelling or touching objects or foodstuffs not normally used on a day-to-day basis within your setting. If in doubt about the suitability of any activity for any child, it is wise to seek the advice and written permission of the parents or carers before embarking, to ensure the well-being of all concerned.

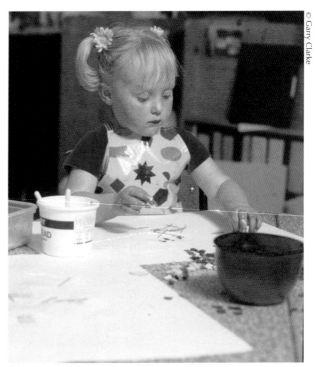
© Garry Clarke

Planning

When planning activities for the children in your setting, it is important to remember that you must cater for a wide range of developmental levels in the group. In addition, each individual child within that group will have constantly changing needs and is not likely to develop at an equal rate in every area of the curriculum.

A thematic approach allows for flexibility within your planning. It caters for those diverse and changing needs by providing a range of activities that are varied and interesting and that constantly stimulate the children's learning. At the same time, it gives a focus for attention, which allows individual children to pursue any special interest that they may have in a particular area for a length of time and in a manner that suits them.

Planning for a progression of ideas

Each chapter of this book deals with a different sense and provides a range of activities that could be introduced over a period of one to two weeks, depending upon the particular interests and skills of the children in your group. The whole book can be covered in this way. If, however, you wish to study 'Senses' as part of a larger overall theme, such as 'Myself' or 'My body', you can dip in and out of the book, selecting a few activities from each chapter to suit the needs of your group. The related songs and rhymes at the end of the book (pages 83–88) can be used to further enhance the children's learning experience.

To assist you with short- and medium-term planning, the 'Further ideas' section at the end of each activity provides starting-points for more related activity ideas, to extend the experience and consolidate the children's learning. There are also theme links to suggest how the activity might lead into another theme, to help you with long-term planning.

Early Learning Goals

The activities within each of the five chapters of this book are arranged to provide progression through the three bands of Stepping Stones that lead to the achievement of the Early Learning Goals. The theme planner on pages 10 and 11 will enable you to readily select activities to suit the various levels of development and particular interests of the children in your setting to cover a range of Stepping Stones within each Area of Learning.

By using continual observation and assessment while completing these activities with the children, you will be able to adapt your plans, as you progress through the theme, to ensure that all the children remain as actively involved as possible throughout.

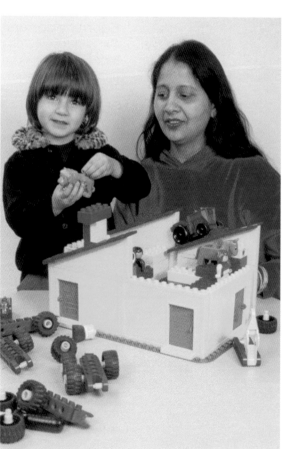

© Derek Cooknell

Foundation Themes
Senses

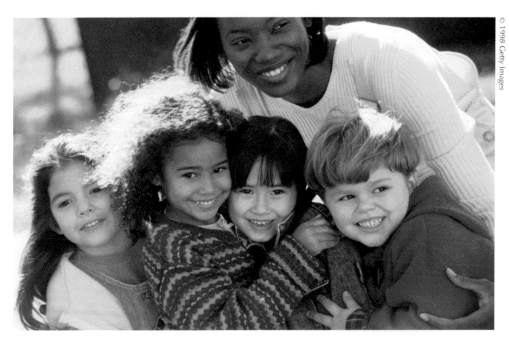

Areas of Learning

As stated in the introduction, the activities within this book cover all Areas of Learning in equal measure. There are 12 activities for each of those Areas and they cover a range of Stepping Stones, progressing from the earliest yellow band level, through the blue and green bands, leading to the Early Learning Goals that the majority of children are expected to achieve by the end of the Foundation Stage. In total, the activities cover Early Learning Goals of four out of the six clusters identified for Personal, social and emotional development; five of the six clusters for Communication, language and literacy; two of the three for Mathematical development; three of the six for Knowledge and understanding of the world; four of the six for Physical development; and all four clusters for Creative development. The theme can, therefore, be used to deliver over two thirds of the Foundation Stage curriculum in an interesting and cohesive manner.

Equal opportunities

The children within your setting will have come from a rich diversity of backgrounds. It is important that you recognise and celebrate this by including provision for every one of them in your planning. The children and their families should feel valued and welcome from the moment they set foot in your building.

The document *Curriculum Guidance for the Foundation Stage* contains information and advice about planning to meet the needs of all children. This includes those with special educational needs (SEN), those who are more able, those with disabilities, boys and girls, and those from different ethnic groups. You may have refugees, asylum seekers and travellers in your setting, and it is important that their needs be considered in your planning, alongside children from different social, cultural or linguistic backgrounds, so that every individual can be offered equal opportunities across the whole curriculum, whatever their background.

The Disability Discrimination Act 1995 has now been extended to cover education, and settings are required to make 'reasonable adjustments', to ensure that disabled children are not at a great disadvantage compared to their able-bodied peers. Practitioners must also ensure that they do not treat disabled children 'less favourably' because of their disability, and this must be taken into account when planning activities for your group. The *Curriculum Guidance for the Foundation Stage* gives advice regarding support and planning for children with SEN or disabilities, to ensure that you are able to provide these children with every opportunity to make the best progress possible, whatever their starting-point.

You should aim to provide a safe, happy, relaxed environment, free from discrimination and harassment, where the children feel that their contributions are valued and respected, and where stereotyping by religion, race, gender or disability is challenged.

You should be aware of the content of various Acts covering the requirements of equal opportunities. These are the Sex Discrimination Act 1975, the Race Relations Act 1976 and the Special Educational Needs and Disability Act 2001, which enabled the Disability Discrimination Act to be extended in September 2002 to cover education. It is also important to consider the requirements of the revised SEN *Code of Practice* during planning.

The activities within this book aim to meet the requirements set out in these documents and should be suitable for most children. However, due to the nature of the theme, some slight adaptations will need to be made in certain situations. For example, materials for use in Chapter 1 will need to be adapted for children with severe sight problems and some activities in Chapter 3 will need adapting to be fully accessible to children with hearing disabilities. It is important that this be taken into account during the planning stage, so that all preparations can be made to have the adapted materials ready before they are required.

Long-, medium- and short-term planning

Effective and efficient planning underpins all that goes on in a setting and is the keystone to providing a lively, interesting and stimulating curriculum for all the children, both on a day-to-day basis and over longer periods of time.

Long-term plans should provide an overview of the various learning experiences and opportunities that will be offered to the children. They should be based on the six Areas of Learning laid down by the QCA and should aim to cover a range of Stepping Stones leading to a variety of Early Learning Goals in each Area. (Refer to the theme planner on pages 10 and 11 to see how the activities in this book can help to cover the Foundation Stage curriculum and many of the Early Learning Goals.) This will ensure the delivery of a broad and balanced curriculum. These plans should be flexible enough to allow you to adapt or introduce specific activities according to the developing and changing needs of the children; therefore, they do not have to contain details of when particular opportunities will be offered. However, they should include the title of a particular theme that you may be working on and the Stepping Stones that you intend to cover at various times within the planned period, as well as any special events that you are planning or visits that you intend to make.

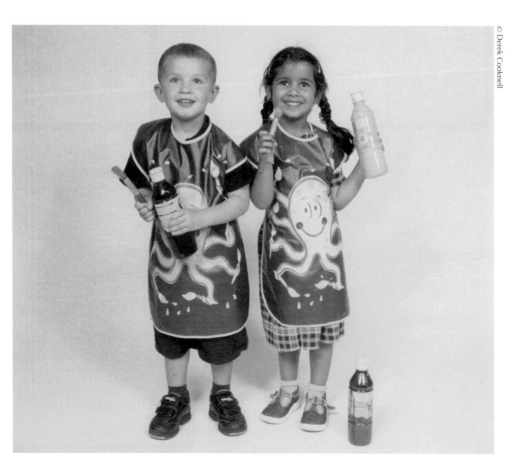

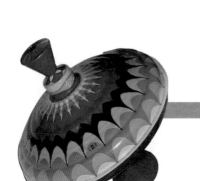

Personal, social and emotional development

ELG clusters	Activity	Page
Dispositions and attitudes	Copycats	16
	Tactile tunnels	35
	In touch with nature	28
	Found it!	47
	Is it this one?	51
	A present for someone special	69
	Fruit salad	78
	Noses	82
Self-confidence and self-esteem	Finger-food buffet	55
Making relationships	Stop, look and listen	24
Behaviour and self-control	Left a bit, stop!	43
	Follow your nose	73

Creative development

ELG clusters	Activity	Page
Exploring media and materials	Look at the colours!	23
	Stir, mix, stretch and pull	38
	It's stopped!	49
	I like sausages!	58
	Rainbow mints	62
Music	Crash, twang, boom!	40
	Pass the bells	77
	Changing sounds	80
Imagination	I smell a boy!	74
Responding to experiences, and expressing and communicating ideas	This is difficult!	21
	Squiggles and swirls	31
	Scented gardens	70

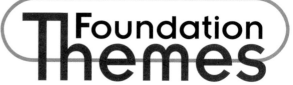

Foundation Themes

Physical development

ELG clusters	Activity	Page
Movement	It's over there!	18
	Hot potato	30
	Feel the shape	36
	Stand up, shake, sit	39
Sense of space	Very carefully	41
	Don't drop it!	76
Using equipment	Be careful!	25
Using tools and materials	Oops!	52
	Easter bonnets	54
	Sensory sand	63
	Spicy pictures	65

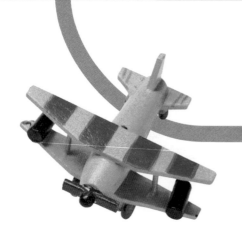

Communication, language and literacy

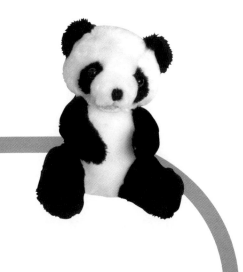

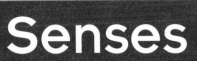

Mathematical development

Knowledge and understanding of the world

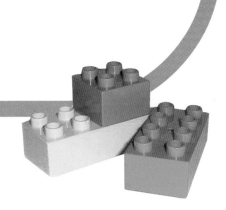

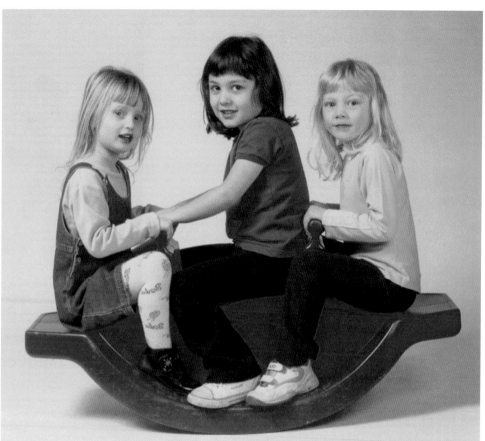

© Derek Cooknell

Medium-term plans provide some 'meat' on the 'bare bones' of the long-term plans and bridge the gap between long- and short-term plans. They should outline the activities that will be offered to cover the Stepping Stones identified in the long-term plans and include details of resources to be used – particularly any that may need to be adapted to make them accessible to any children with special needs. It might be useful at this stage to include contact details of any outside agencies that may be able to provide specialist equipment, resources or expertise to aid the efficient delivery of the planned activities to those children. A member of staff can then be allocated the task of contacting these agencies and arranging any necessary meetings or the acquisition or adaptation of the available resources prior to the short-term planning stage. Medium-term plans should also include details regarding the organisation, groupings and teaching strategies that will be employed to deliver the planned curriculum and to identify the assessment opportunities that will arise. The plans should provide a clear and practical guide of what is to be done and when, and should be readily accessible to all staff members.

Short-term plans provide further details of the activities that are being offered and how they are to be carried out. They should contain clear information regarding the role of the adults – including any parent helpers – and detail any adjustments that will need to be made to cater for children with different needs. It is important at this stage that any specialist advice or equipment gathered at the medium-term planning stage be checked and consolidated and that all staff be fully briefed about how to make use of it to the best advantage. Short-term plans should also include specific details, such as the vocabulary that is to be used or introduced and how links can be made to other Areas of Learning or to other related activities that can be or have been carried out. They should cover all six Areas of Learning and identify how assessments are to be conducted and recorded. You should draw up short-term plans on a daily or weekly basis, so that you can take into account any changing conditions or circumstances within the setting and highlight any amendments that will need to be made at any particular time.

All plans should be clear, concise and informative, yet remain easy to complete, so that you and other staff members do not need to spend undue amounts of time on them. They should make your lives easier, not more difficult!

Assessment

Children arrive at pre-school settings from all walks of life and with a multitude of diverse experiences behind them. Assessment plays an important role in working with children, since it helps practitioners to ascertain at what stage each child is developmentally and enables them to plan activities accordingly.

The importance of assessment

The *Curriculum Guidance for the Foundation Stage* sets out the Stepping Stones that lead to the achievement of the Early Learning Goals for each Area of Learning in a roughly hierarchical order. Few children will progress steadily through these Stepping Stones in that order, and few will make equal progress across all Areas of Learning. It is important, therefore, that you keep track of individual progress in all areas of the curriculum, through regular assessment. For example, some children may appear to have achieved the later Stepping Stones and yet still lack confidence in some of the earlier ones. Regular and systematic assessment will help you to identify these gaps in learning and enable you to adapt or amend your planned activities to cater for the diverse and changing needs of each child in your care.

Assessment is not just important for the individual child, but also for groups of children, particularly, but not solely, in the area of Personal, social and emotional development, where interaction between individuals is a key issue. Close observations and regular assessments of a particular group, or groups, of children will help you to identify any potential problems in their initial stages. This means that you will be able to take remedial action before things get out of hand. Being aware of how various groups of children interact is important across the entire curriculum, since it can influence the way that you organise both your setting and the activities within it.

Methods of assessment

Assessment should not be an arduous task that consumes vast amounts of time and energy – if it were, it would do more harm than good. It should be built into the daily routine, so that it becomes an automatic part of the working day. Evidence can be collected and recorded with varying degrees of formality, but it is important to ensure that written records are readily accessible to all staff members and regularly updated, and provide a true picture of the individual child in all areas of development. It is also important to ensure that assessments, whether formal or informal, remain focused, in order for them to provide the sort of useful information that will assist you in your planning.

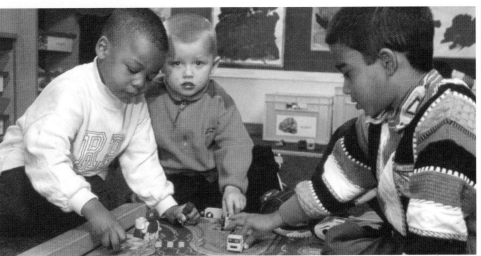

© Derek Cooknell

Assessments can be conducted in a variety of ways and in many different situations. Practitioners can be silent observers, watching but not intervening in the child's play; they can converse with the child, to find out more about what they are thinking or feeling; or they can become an interactive member of the whole group, either to steer the activity in a particular direction or to follow where the children lead. There are various ways to record your observations: you can use a pen and notepad to scribble notes, either during the observation or as soon as possible after it has been carried out; you can set up a tape recorder to gather evidence, which can be reviewed at leisure when time allows; you can use a still camera to record evidence of a child's achievement, which might otherwise go unnoticed; or you can make a video, which can be shared with the child, their parents or carers, or other practitioners.

Formal assessment

In addition to your ongoing assessment, in the children's final term of the Foundation Stage, you and your staff will be completing individual *Foundation Stage Profile* documents. These will record the progress that each child has made. There will also be times when it may be necessary to conduct more formal assessments. You may need to obtain precise and detailed information about a particular aspect of a child's development in order to ascertain how best to help that child – for example, if they have specific learning difficulties, behavioural problems or a physical disability. In such cases, it is important for practitioners to decide exactly what evidence they need, how best to collect it and to devise a systematic way of recording it, before they begin the assessment.

Gaining evidence of skills

Although young children learn at different rates and pick up some skills more easily than others, they all need to practise those skills many times in order to become confident and proficient in their use. Not only are they constantly acquiring new skills, but they are also learning how and when to use them. So what they appear to do with ease on one particular day, in one particular situation, they will often struggle with the following day, in a different situation. It is important, therefore, that all practitioners, when assessing those skills in individual children, gather their evidence over a period of time and select activities that will allow the child to use those skills in a variety of situations and with varying degrees of support and encouragement.

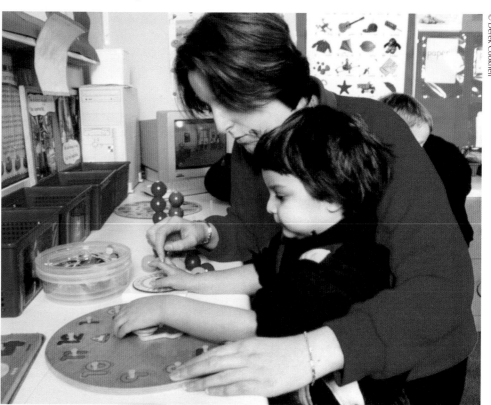

© Derek Cooknell

Chapter 1

Sight

This chapter offers activities that encourage children to express and communicate their thoughts and feelings, solve practical problems and ask questions about why things happen and how things work. It also gives them opportunities to imagine and re-create roles and experiences, and to use a range of tools and equipment.

Changing patterns

Group size
Four children.

What you need
Kaleidoscopes; mirror card; sticky tape; guillotine; pencil; ruler.

Preparation
Use the guillotine to cut the card into various lengths and widths, no smaller than 15cm x 6cm.

What to do
Look at the kaleidoscopes together and discuss how they work. Tell the children that you are going to show them how to make one of their own. Select a piece of card and explain that it must be folded into a triangular tube with the mirror on the inside.

Demonstrate how to place the card, mirror-side down, with about a third of it overhanging the edge of the table. Fold it down along the edge of the table to get a sharp, straight crease. Turn the card around and repeat along its other side to give two parallel creases, dividing the card into three roughly equal sections. Count these with the children before bringing the outer edges of the card together and taping them securely to make a mirror-lined triangular prism. Invite each child in turn to put the tube close to their eye and look through it as they slowly scan the room.

Help each child to make a kaleidoscope. (It is not essential that the sides of their triangles be exactly the same length, nor that the edges of the kaleidoscope be precisely parallel, since any irregularities will merely produce different effects, but it is important to seal the join securely to exclude light along the length of the tube.) Invite the children to use their kaleidoscopes to explore various objects around the room. As they work, talk to them about what they can see and encourage them to explain what they think might be happening. Discuss the differences between their kaleidoscopes and the commercially produced ones.

Stepping Stone
Show an interest in why things happen and how things work.

Early Learning Goal
Ask questions about why things happen and how things work.

Support and extension
Using a pencil and ruler, draw guidelines for younger children to fold along. Ask older children to invite a friend and instruct them how to make their own kaleidoscope.

Home partnership
Let the children take their kaleidoscopes home for further investigation. Encourage them to share their discoveries with the group next session.

Further ideas
♦ Investigate a collection of everyday objects with reflective surfaces, including kettles, saucepans, spoons, aluminium foil and cans.
♦ Set up the interactive display 'Patterns' on page 79.

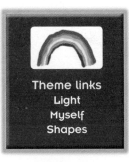

Theme links
Light
Myself
Shapes

Copycats

Stepping Stone
Show confidence in linking up with others for support and guidance.

Early Learning Goal
Be confident to try new activities.

Group size
Up to eight children, in pairs.

What you need
Paper; collage materials; writing tools.

Preparation
Ensure that all the children have had some experience of working freely with similar materials before embarking on this activity.

What to do
Gather the group together and explain that they are going to work in pairs to make two pictures that look the same. Explain to the children that they must take turns to tell each other what to put on the picture next and where to place it. Then discuss being fair and taking turns.

Give each child a sheet of paper and invite them to write their name on the back, before they find partners and set to work. Observe the pairs of children and be ready to remind them that their pictures should look the same. Ensure that the children remember to take turns to lead the activity, and remind them to use their eyes very carefully to see where their partner is placing a piece and to check that it corresponds to their own.

Show the children how to put their pictures close together to check that they match and help them to decide what to do if they do not! When a pair of children decide that their picture is complete, ask them to look at it carefully to make sure that they are satisfied with it. Do they both look the same? Is there anything more that they wish to add?

When the creations are dry, display them randomly on a board and ask the group to try to spot the matching pairs and to say how they know that they match.

Support and extension
It may be necessary to physically demonstrate the activity to very young children, to help them understand exactly how to take turns. Challenge older children to stick to a particular theme or introduce a rule such as, 'Use a maximum of three colours'.

Home partnership
Ask the children to find identical pairs at home, for example, cushions, socks or curtains, and to draw a picture of them to show to the group.

Further ideas
♦ Play 'Follow-my-leader' by running around in pairs, one behind the other, and, on a given signal, running the opposite way, with the second child as leader.
♦ Sing the song 'Can you?' on the photocopiable sheet on page 86 with the children.
♦ Tell a group story by taking turns to add an element, using pictures as a stimulus.

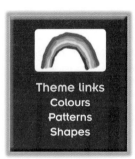

Theme links
Colours
Patterns
Shapes

Foundation Themes
Senses

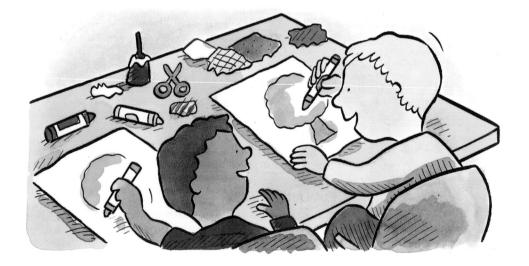

How many now?

Group size
Up to eight children.

What you need
Unbreakable mirrors of different sizes; small items, such as buttons, counters or play people; drawing and writing materials.

What to do

Gather the group together around a table and look at the mirrors. Talk about what you see when you look in a mirror and lead the children to realise that whatever size a mirror is, it will always reflect just one of each object put in front of it.

Provide each child with a mirror, placing one button in front of it. Ask how many buttons they can see. Give them another button or two and ask them, in turn, to count their buttons and to say the total.

Next, invite the children to experiment with the materials to find various totals, encouraging them to explain what they are doing as they work. Have writing materials close at hand and invite interested children to record some of their experiments in numbers, words or pictures.

Finally, again, give each child a mirror and just one button. Challenge them to find a way of positioning the button and the mirror so that only one button can be seen in total. If no solution is found, tell the group that you will leave the equipment out for them to try again whenever they like. Once a solution has been found, gather the group together and invite the solver to demonstrate their method.

Support and extension

Ensure that younger children have time for unstructured experiential play with mirrors, before expecting them to complete this activity. Introduce the word 'double' to older or more able children and encourage them to use a mirror to find doubles of numbers up to a total of ten.

Home partnership

Ask parents and carers to help their children to count how many people are in the house, gather them in front of the mirror and count again, to find out how many real and reflected people there are altogether, and then to record the activity pictorially to share with the group.

Further ideas

♦ Draw half-pictures and use mirrors to make them whole.
♦ Hinge two mirrors together with sticky tape and experiment with increasing and decreasing amounts of objects seen by changing the angle.

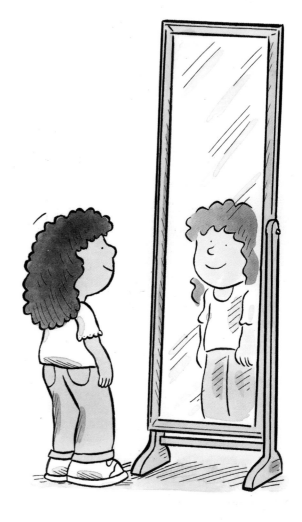

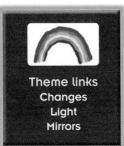

Theme links
Changes
Light
Mirrors

Foundation Themes
Senses

It's over there!

Stepping Stone
Negotiate space successfully when playing racing and chasing games with other children.

Group size
Whole group.

What you need
A large defined space; large coloured discs or sheets of paper, two of each colour.

Preparation
Position one disc of each colour around the edge of the space, so that it can be seen clearly from a distance.

What to do
Ask the group to spread out around the space and practise walking and stopping at a given signal. Then

Early Learning Goal
Move with confidence, imagination and in safety.

invite the children to practise *running* and stopping, reminding them that they must watch carefully where they are going, so as not to bump into one another. Now encourage them to practise running in various directions, depending on where you point and, again, stopping at a given signal.

After a few minutes, stop the group and ask them if they have noticed anything around the edge of the room (the coloured discs). Show them the spare discs, talk about the colours and ensure that most children can match each spare disc to its partner around the edge. Explain to the children that when you hold up a disc they must run to the matching colour and stand still.

Play the game several times before gathering the children together to bring the activity to a close. Talk about what they have been doing and ask them to tell you why their eyes were important during the activity (for finding the right colours and avoiding obstacles while running).

Finish by looking at the discs one by one, naming the colour and asking the children to use their eyes to spy an object of the same colour in the room.

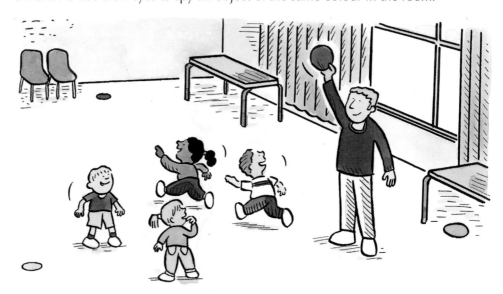

Support and extension
Help younger or less confident children to find a friend to run with. Introduce action words with older children, so that they 'hop', 'skip', 'jump', 'gallop' or 'roll' to the specified area.

Home partnership
Encourage parents and carers to play 'Colour I spy' with their children on the way home or on any journey.

Further ideas
♦ Give the children strips of different-coloured crêpe paper and encourage them to run freely in a large open space, indoors or outdoors, to make the paper stream out behind them. This is fun outside on windy days.
♦ Place marker discs or cones randomly around the room and practise dodging and weaving between them.

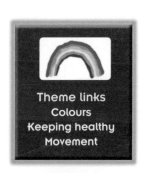

Theme links
Colours
Keeping healthy
Movement

Foundation Themes
Senses

Look what's happened!

Stepping Stone
Talk about what is seen and
what is happening.

Early Learning Goal
Look closely at
similarities, differences,
patterns and change.

Group size
Up to six children.

What you need
Card; short, thin,
round sticks, or
strong drinking
straws; drawing
materials; sticky
tape; glue.

Preparation
Cut the card
into pieces,
approximately 10cm
x 7cm, two for each
child. Then make
a demonstration
model following the
instructions in 'What
to do'.

What to do
Gather the children together and look at each side of your model, talking about what you can see. Ask the children to watch the picture carefully while you spin it, by turning the stick rapidly between your palms.

Encourage the children to talk about what they saw and what they think is happening to the two pictures, then invite them to make similar spinners of their own. Provide each child with a piece of card and ask them to draw a picture of a birdcage, making it as large as possible, so as to fill the page.

Give the children a second piece each and ask them to draw a colourful bird. Help each child to tape a stick to the back of one picture, so that there is at least 7cm protruding from the bottom of the picture. Glue the two pictures back to back.

Once the glue is dry, demonstrate how to rub the palms together to make the pictures spin, so that the bird appears to be inside the cage. Again, encourage the children to explain what they think is happening.

Support and extension
Younger children may need considerable help and practice to perfect the spinning of the pictures. Encourage older children to invent other pairs of pictures, such as flowers in vases, apples on trees, noses on clowns and so on.

Home partnership
Let the children take home their spinners, and encourage parents and carers to ask them to try to explain how they made these and how they work.

Further ideas
♦ Investigate other optical illusions, such as those in *Eye Magic* by Sarah Hewetson and Phil Jacobs (Western Publishing Company).
♦ Use reflective silver card to make a set of curved mirrors that each give a different effect when looked into, and invite the children to investigate for themselves by bending, folding or twisting the card.

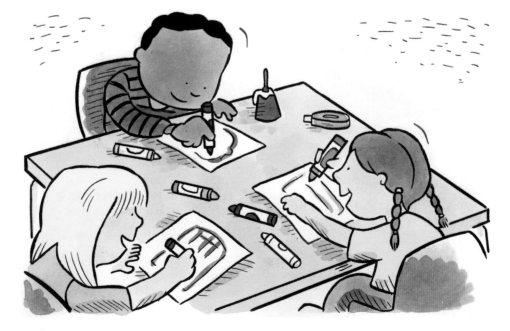

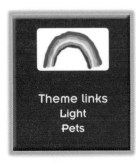

Theme links
Light
Pets

Foundation
Themes
Senses

Eyes can...

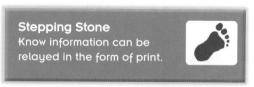

Stepping Stone
Know information can be relayed in the form of print.

Early Learning Goal
Know that print carries meaning and, in English, is read from left to right and top to bottom.

Group size
Whole group initially, then up to four children at a time.

What you need
The rhyme 'My eyes' on the photocopiable sheet on page 83; coloured A2 paper; A3 paper; A5 paper; stapler; writing, drawing and craft materials.

Preparation
Photocopy the rhyme on to A3 paper. Fold and staple three sheets of coloured A2 paper to make a book called 'My eyes'.

What to do
Position the rhyme so that everyone can see it and point to the words as you read it. Then say it again, this time talking about each action and inviting the children to join in.

Next, suggest that it might be fun to make the rhyme into a big book for everyone to share. Ask for volunteers to start, while the rest of the group follow other activities. Read the first line again with the children and challenge them to make pictures, on A5 paper, of themselves with an eye that can wink. Invite them to cut out their pictures and paste them on the first page of the book.

Then, write 'My eyes can wink' under the pictures and read the words with the children. Send each child to fetch a friend to continue the activity.

Repeat with the new group, this time working on the second line of the rhyme. Continue in this way until the rhyme is complete and the book is full.

Finally, gather the whole group together and go through the finished book, reading the words and doing the actions. Leave the book accessible for the children to read for themselves freely.

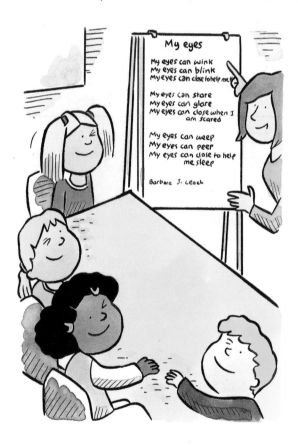

Support and extension
Help very young children to give expression to their drawings, by talking them through the process, step by step. Encourage older children to write the text themselves.

Home partnership
Ask the children to bring in from home old newspapers and magazines containing faces, so that they can cut out pairs of eyes to decorate the cover of the book.

Further ideas
♦ Make large flash cards of action words or directions and play games by reading the words and doing the actions, for example, 'look up', 'wink' and 'blink'.
♦ Play 'Hunt the word' using pairs of word cards, hiding one, giving the other to a child and challenging them to find its duplicate.

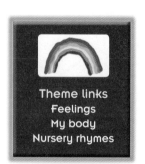

Theme links
Feelings
My body
Nursery rhymes

Foundation
Themes
Senses

This is difficult!

Stepping Stone
Talk about personal intentions, describing what they were trying to do.

Early Learning Goal
Express and communicate their ideas, thoughts and feelings by using a widening range of materials.

Group size
Four children.

What you need
Play dough; cardboard box for each child; scissors or sharp knife (adult use).

Preparation
Cut two hand holes in one side of each box.

What to do
Give the play dough to the children and invite them to make it into different shapes or models. Talk to them as they work and encourage them to explain what they are doing and what they hope to achieve. After several minutes challenge them to make specific items, for example, a flower, a person, a snail and so on.

Discuss the finished products and how they were made and congratulate the children on being so clever. Then challenge them to repeat the activity without looking at what they are doing! Put their latest model to one side and give each child a box containing a fresh piece of dough. Invite them to put their hands through the holes and work blind to produce an item like the one that they have just put aside, without referring to it. Again, encourage them to explain what they are doing as they work. Once they think that their model is finished, invite them to take it carefully out of the box and compare it with the original.

To close the activity, gather a small group of children together and ask the artists to show their models and explain what they have been doing. Leave the boxes and play dough accessible and suggest that other children might like to have a go themselves some time.

Support and extension
Put younger children's first models on top of their boxes, so that each child can refer to their model as they work blind. Encourage older children to challenge each other to produce more complex models as they become more adept at working blind.

Home partnership
Explain to parents and carers what you have been doing and encourage them to challenge their children to draw pictures or build towers without looking.

Further ideas
♦ Display the children's paintings, drawings and models in an 'Artists' corner', adding a few explanatory or descriptive words from the artists about their work.
♦ Fill shallow trays with different materials, such as fine gravel, cornflour paste, lentils or cooked spaghetti, and invite the children to explore them with spoons, forks or fingers, talking as they work.

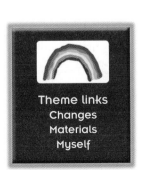

Theme links
Changes
Materials
Myself

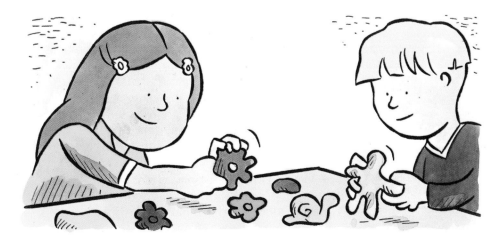

Foundation
Themes
Senses

Where next?

Stepping Stone
Describe a simple journey.

Early Learning Goal
Use everyday words to describe position.

Group size
Pairs of children.

What you need
Space indoors or outdoors to set up a trail; coloured card; scissors; writing materials; Blu-Tack.

Preparation
Make sets of six triangles, squares, rectangles and circles, numbered 1 to 6, and a set of directional arrows.

What to do

Give a set of shapes to the first pair of children and explain that they are going to make a trail for their friends to follow. Tell them that they will need to put the shapes and numbers in the correct order, and an arrow to show which way to go next.

Help the children to decide which number they should begin with and where to position it. Use Blu-Tack to stick the shape on to a suitable object and invite the children to decide which way to go next. Secure an arrow beneath the shape, ensuring that it is pointing in the agreed direction. Continue to lay the trail until all six shapes are in position, along with their directional arrows.

Return to base and ask the children to select two friends to follow their trail. The trail-setters remain at base while the adult accompanies the followers. Stop at each shape as it is spotted and talk about where the children have come from and where the arrow is telling them to go next.

Once all the shapes and arrows are collected, return to base and invite the followers to describe their journey to the setters. Ask the followers and setters to swap roles and carry out the activity again using a different set of shapes and a different route.

Repeat with other children in the group.

Support and extension

Use large, brightly coloured shapes with very young children and place them at child height. Challenge older children to set more than one trail at a time, letting the different routes converge and diverge at will.

Home partnership

Invite the children to describe journeys within their home, for example, from the front door to their bedroom, from the garden to the bathroom, from the kitchen to the dustbin, and so on.

Further ideas

♦ Ask the children to take turns to hide an object and direct their friend to it verbally, by saying, for example, 'It's under something blue', 'It's behind a chair that's near the door' and so on.
♦ Invite a child who lives close to the setting to lead the group (with you in charge) on a walk to their house, and ask someone else to lead you back.
♦ Make a copy of the photocopiable sheet 'Shape trails' on page 89 for each child so that they can practise following shape trails and writing numbers in order.

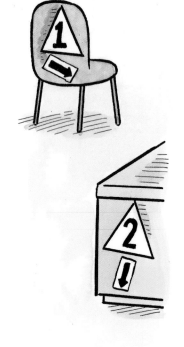

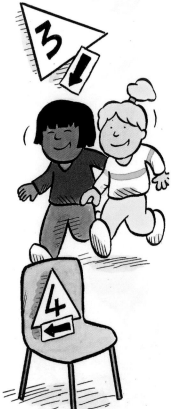

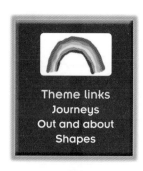

Theme links
Journeys
Out and about
Shapes

Foundation
Themes
Senses

Look at the colours!

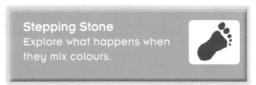
Early Learning Goal
Explore colour, texture, shape, form and space in two or three dimensions.

Group size
Up to six children.

What you need
Clear plastic, acetate or Cellophane; coloured tissue; coloured acetate or Cellophane; strong glue that dries clear; scissors.

What to do
Show the children the coloured materials and invite them to put them together, hold them up to the light and look through them. Ask them what they notice.

Once they have had several minutes to experiment with the different colours, introduce the clear plastic and the glue. Explain that they are going to make pictures through which light can shine, to make new and exciting colours. Invite the children to explain how this might be done. Lead them to realise that new colours are formed when different colours overlap, and that different depths of colour are achieved when the same colours are layered. Demonstrate this with some of the materials. Have scissors accessible, so that the children can adapt shapes and sizes to suit their designs. Suggest that brushing a thin layer of glue on to a section of the clear plastic and gently laying the coloured paper on top is probably the best way to avoid too much glue and torn tissue paper.

Leave the pictures to dry before displaying them on a window and gathering the group around to admire and comment upon the designs and colours.

Support and extension
Use only acetate or Cellophane with very young children, as tissue paper tends to disintegrate in less dexterous hands! Encourage older children to think out, and perhaps sketch, their designs before they begin, and to look at them carefully when they have finished to see if they need any amendments or additions.

Home partnership
Ask parents and carers for any discarded net curtains and dye them different colours for the children to experiment with colour-mixing on a large scale.

Further ideas
♦ Add a few drops of food colouring to the water tray and use different-coloured transparent containers to create different effects when pouring and tipping.
♦ Provide the children with palettes and ask them to mix their own paint colours without spoiling the main paint pots.

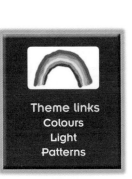

Theme links
Colours
Light
Patterns

Foundation
Themes
Senses

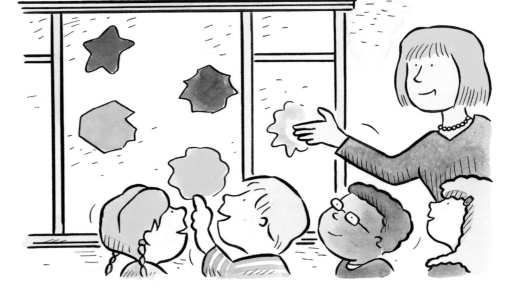

Stop, look and listen

Stepping Stone
Value and contribute to own well-being and self-control.

Group size
Whole group.

What you need
Posters or large photographs of a range of road signs and signals, such as traffic lights, pedestrian crossings, children crossing signs, crossing-patrol lollipops and Belisha beacons; paper; clipboards; pens.

What to do
Tell the group that you have some pictures of things that you have seen when you were out walking and you wonder if they can help you to decide what they are. Look at the first picture together and invite the children to say what it might be.

Talk about what the picture shows, where you might find such an object and what it might be for. Discuss its importance in keeping people safe near roads and explain that signs and signals are all around us and we must remember to pay attention to them. Talk about what might happen if motorists did not take notice of a red light, or pedestrians ignored the 'little red man'.

Explain that you are going for a walk to see how many signs and signals you can find in your locality and remind the children to walk sensibly, using their eyes the whole time. Take clipboards and pens with you on your walk and suggest to the children that they might like to sketch some of the signs that they see, to help them remember what they look like and where they were.

When you return, recall your route and invite volunteers to show their sketches, talk about what they saw, and find their sign among your posters or photographs.

Finally, display posters and sketches alongside one another, with a brief summary of your walk and what you saw.

Support and extension
Take very young children out in groups of only four or six, accompanied by at least two adults. Encourage older children to improve their sketches once they get back to the setting, and to add a few descriptive words.

Home partnership
Ask parents and carers to help their children to spot road signs and signals when out and about, particularly unusual ones such as the one showing ducks crossing.

Further ideas
♦ Invite your local community police officer in to talk to the group about personal safety.
♦ Set up the role-play area with pedestrian crossings or traffic-lights to practise the procedure for crossing roads safely.

Early Learning Goal
Work as part of a group or class, taking turns and sharing fairly, understanding that there needs to be agreed values and codes of behaviour for groups of people, including adults and children, to work together harmoniously.

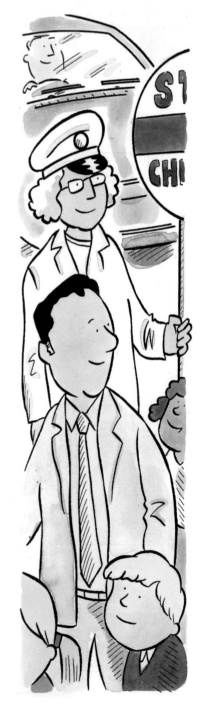

Theme links
Journeys
Out and about
People who help us

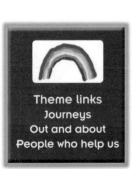

Foundation
Themes
Senses

Be careful!

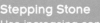
Group size
Four children.

What you need
Softwood, 30cm x 30cm; screw-in L-shaped cup hooks; sticky labels; pens; very thick card; thin wire; strong scissors and staple gun (adult use); somewhere to hang the finished board; straws or tally-sticks.

Preparation
Make several card hoops by cutting out 7cm diameter circles and removing 5cm circles from their centres. Make a loop of wire and staple it to one corner of the wood square, so that it can hang diagonally.

What to do
Tell the children that they are going to make a game to see how clever they are at throwing. Introduce the square of wood with the hanging loop and then show them the hoops. Ask for suggestions of what else you might need to make these things into a game.

Now show the children the hooks and point out that each has a screw at one end. Demonstrate how to screw a hook into the board, positioning it in the centre. Invite the children to take turns to screw a hook into a different corner, reminding them to think about which way up they have to place it.

Suggest that it might make the game more exciting if you could score points, and invite each child to write a number on a label and stick it by their hook.

Finally, suspend the board at a suitable height on a convenient wall and let the children take turns to throw the hoops and try to get them on the hooks.

Support and extension
Help younger children to keep their scores by using straws or tally-sticks. Encourage older children to keep their scores mentally.

Home partnership
Ask parents and carers to help their children to invent throwing games, using balls, paper plates or scrunched-up paper to aim at targets such as buckets, bowls or suspended hoops.

Further ideas
♦ Set up a variety of skills-practising games, such as dribbling balls between cones, throwing balls through hoops, rolling balls into arches cut into cardboard boxes, or juggling with chiffon squares.
♦ Use cardboard tubes of varying lengths to make lightweight hockey sticks, croquet mallets, baseball bats or golf clubs, to use with small sponge balls.

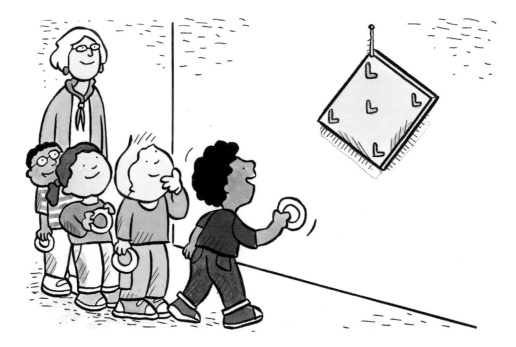

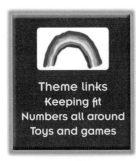

Theme links
Keeping fit
Numbers all around
Toys and games

Foundation Themes
Senses

Do you have an appointment?

Group size
Six to eight children.

What you need
The photocopiable sheet 'Eye chart' on page 90; card; Blu-Tack; frames of old spectacles or sun-glasses; chairs; desk; writing equipment; old diary; small offcuts of card; telephone; white jackets or shirts; unbreakable mirrors.

Preparation
Copy the photocopiable sheet twice on to card and laminate each sheet. Affix one copy to a suitable surface at child's eye level, and cut off the strip of symbols at the bottom of the other copy.

What to do
Talk to the group about what an optician is and why we need to have regular eye tests. Encourage the children to relate any personal experiences to the group and to explain what happened during their last visit.

Look at the equipment together and talk about what it is for: the diary, telephone and small cards for making and remembering appointments; the white jackets for the optician and assistants; the frames for choosing a suitable style of glasses; and the eye chart for testing the eyes.

Show the children the strip of symbols and explain that they are for helping the person who is having their eyes tested. Instead of naming the symbol that they see, they can find a matching one from the strip to show to the optician.

Play alongside the children as their game develops, modelling appropriate behaviour and vocabulary, and extending their play without taking over.

At the end of the session, encourage the children to tidy the area and leave it ready for another time.

Support and extension
Support younger or less confident children by role-playing a parent or friend and accompanying them to 'the optician's'. Encourage older children to fill out appointment cards realistically, with the name, day, date and time clearly shown.

Home partnership
Invite parents and carers to donate plastic frames of old spectacles and sun-glasses to add to your collection.

Further ideas
♦ Extend the children's experiences by sometimes modelling the role-play area on less familiar environments, such as a railway station, a museum or an art exhibition.
♦ Provide opportunities for the children to develop their imaginative play by equipping the role-play area with items such as huge cardboard boxes, lengths of fabric and building blocks.

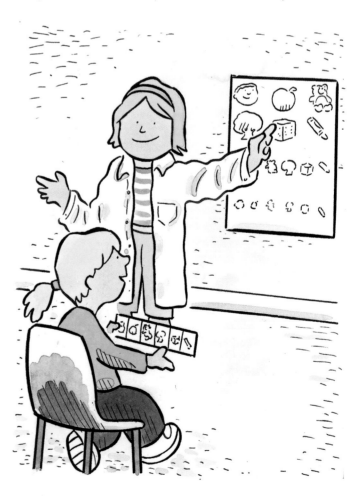

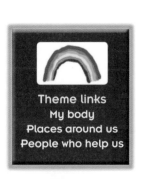

Theme links
My body
Places around us
People who help us

Foundation
Themes
Senses

Chapter 2

Touch

The activities in this chapter encourage the children to literally take the world in their hands and explore texture, shape and form while practising a variety of cross-curricular skills, such as counting, building and constructing, and running and dodging. They also provide opportunities to investigate objects and materials and to enjoy the spoken word.

Egg and eggshells

Group size
Up to six children.

What you need
Clean, roughly crushed eggshells; whole egg; fabric offcuts; strong glue; brushes; scissors; large sheet of paper for each child; other art and craft materials as desired; typed copy of 'Humpty Dumpty' (Traditional) for each child.

Preparation
Gather the group together and sing 'Humpty Dumpty'. Talk about the words of the song and what they mean, before suggesting to the children that they each make their own Humpty, using real eggshells.

What to do
Give each child a large sheet of paper and a copy of 'Humpty Dumpty'. Ask them to paste their rhyme either at the top or the bottom of their paper. Then read the words through together.

Carefully pass the egg around the group, letting the children feel it. Talk about how delicate it is and what would happen if it fell off a wall. Invite the children to feel the eggshells and compare them to the whole egg.

Help each child to draw a large oval on their paper, leaving room for legs at the bottom. Demonstrate how to spread glue on the upper half of the oval and sprinkle eggshells on to it, gently pressing down any odd pieces where necessary.

Invite the children to feel the fabrics and to each choose which they would like for Humpty's clothes, then help them to cut it to fit the lower half of the oval. Add arms, legs and facial features, using whatever materials you have available.

Finally, read through the rhyme together once more and comment upon what a good job everyone has made of putting Humpty together again, even though the King's men had not been able to manage it!

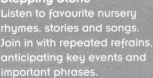
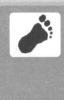

Stepping Stone
Listen to favourite nursery rhymes, stories and songs. Join in with repeated refrains, anticipating key events and important phrases.

Early Learning Goal
Enjoy listening to and using spoken and written language, and readily turn to it in their play and learning.

Support and extension
Prepare the materials for very young children by drawing the oval and cutting out arms, legs and semi-ovals of fabric. Encourage older children to write the rhyme themselves, rather than using a printed copy.

Home partnership
Encourage the children to read their rhyme through with their families when they take Humpty home.

Further ideas
♦ Make props and use them to act out various nursery rhymes in the role-play area.
♦ Record yourself on a tape reading a favourite story, for the children to listen to as they turn the pages of the corresponding book.

Theme links
Materials
Nursery rhymes
Shapes

In touch with nature

Stepping Stone
Have a strong exploratory impulse.

Early Learning Goal
Continue to be interested, excited and motivated to learn.

Group size
Up to six children.

What you need
An outdoor environment.

Preparation
Explain to the children that you are going to go outside to explore the area and that it is important that you all stay together and that they listen to you very carefully.

Check for allergies, such as hay fever, before you begin, and adapt your route accordingly.

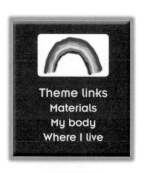

Theme links
Materials
My body
Where I live

What to do
Go outside and gather around a suitable feature, such as a tree. Invite the children to close their eyes, touch the trunk of the tree and talk about what it feels like. Encourage them to touch with their fingertips, palms, backs of hands and even cheeks. Ask them what it feels like to hug the tree. Explain to them that you are going to be touching other objects and plants outside, but that they must not touch anything without first asking an adult, because some things might be dangerous.

Explore the area together, trying to experience a wide range of items. For example, you could touch rough and smooth stones, feathers, dandelion seeds, holly leaves, daisy petals, wet grass and so on. For children with allergies, concentrate on the constructed environment, including rough tarmac, smooth paving slabs, wooden fences and brick walls.

As you explore, collect any suitable objects to take back inside for further investigation later. When you return to your setting, ensure that everyone washes their hands thoroughly.

Finally, gather the group together and talk about what you have been doing. Invite individuals to describe what they enjoyed or disliked the most. Display the collected objects, adding some descriptive words chosen by the children, and leave them to be explored freely during subsequent sessions.

Support and extension
Help younger children to experience delicate items, such as dandelion seeds, by brushing the object against their hands or cheeks rather than trying to hold it. Encourage older children to think of similes to describe things, for example, 'It's as soft as cat's fur'.

Home partnership
Encourage the children to bring in something textured from home, such as sandpaper, a furry slipper or a rubber glove, to make a feely display.

Further ideas
♦ Fill a bowl with cooked spaghetti, cover it with black plastic, make slits in it with a knife and invite the children to explore the bowl by dipping their hands through these.
♦ Put fine gravel in a shallow tray and invite the children to make various patterns in it with their fingers.

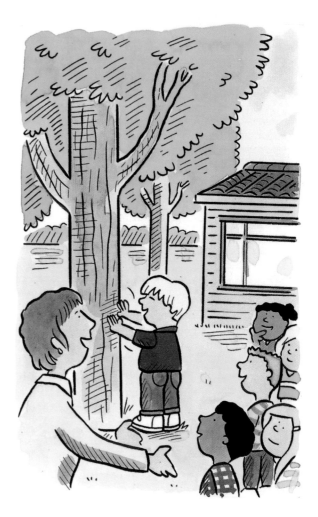

What shall we make?

Early Learning Goal
Build and construct with a wide range of objects, selecting appropriate resources, and adapting their work where necessary.

Group size
Up to eight children.

What you need
A variety of construction materials with different textures, such as corrugated card or plastic, smooth laminated wood, fibreboard, plywood, block foam, hardboard, cardboard of various thicknesses and cardboard tubes; fabrics; pens; paper.

Preparation
Ensure that all materials are safe, with no splinters or very rough edges.

What to do
Invite the group to explore the materials freely and observe them as they work. Encourage the children to talk about what they are doing, and be ready to help with suggestions if they become frustrated in their efforts to build a chosen object.

Talk to them about the feel of the various materials, asking them questions such as, 'Does the thin card feel strong enough to make a bridge?', 'What other material might be more suitable?' and so on. Discuss with the children the wisdom of stacking heavy materials to make precariously high towers. Encourage them to think about the suitability of the chosen material *before* putting it to use. Then ask them to consider what it would feel like to drive over a road, or go down a slide, made of corrugated card.

Once a structure has been completed to a child's satisfaction, draw the group together to admire it and talk about the materials used. Give the builder a chance to say whether they are satisfied with the result or whether they think that it could be improved upon next time. Finally, talk about the available materials and invite the children to suggest others that might be useful additions in the future.

Support and extension
With very young children, be ready to intervene as they may try to build dangerously unsound structures using unsuitably heavy materials. Encourage older children to draw plans of their constructions before they build them and to adapt them to fit the available materials.

Home partnership
Ask parents and carers to donate offcuts of wood, card and fabric to add to your stocks and encourage them to be on the look-out for less common items, such as huge cardboard boxes, wool cones or carpet tubes, which you may find useful.

Further ideas
♦ Paint empty tissue boxes with a mixture of paint and sand for realistically textured building bricks.
♦ Make a giant dolls' house, using large cardboard boxes painted on the outside and decorated on the inside with end-rolls of wallpaper and offcuts of carpet.

Theme links
Homes
People's jobs
Where I live

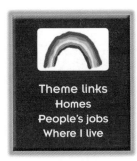

Foundation Themes
Senses

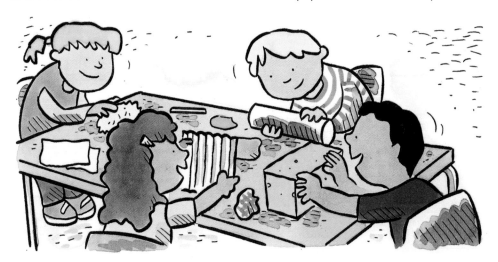

Hot potato

Group size
Whole group.

What you need
Beanbags or
small balls; large,
defined, open
space.

What to do

Explain that you are going to play
'Hot potato'. Talk to the children
about what it might feel like to hold a hot potato. Conclude that if someone handed
you one, you would want to get rid of it as soon as possible.

Show the children the beanbags and explain that they are going to be the hot
potatoes, so, if they are given one, they must run as fast as they can and give it to
someone else before it burns their fingers. Say that everyone else in the room must
stand still and only those with the potatoes must run.

Practise with just one potato at first: give it to a child, who then must run, give it
to someone else and stand still again to watch the next child run with the potato.
Remind the runners to look where they are going, so that they do not bump into
anyone, and to give the potato only to someone who is standing still. Once the
children understand what is expected of them, introduce more beanbags until the
room is full of frantic bodies rushing hither and thither!

After a few minutes, stop the game and feel a potato. Announce that it is not
so hot now, so there is no need to run so fast, and continue the game at a jogging
pace. Then, after another minute or two, stop the game and pronounce the potatoes
cool enough to allow the carriers to walk. Finish the game by deeming the potatoes
too cold to play with.

Support and extension

Very young children may be
overwhelmed by the frenetic
activity at first, so calm it
down a little by facing inwards
in a circle, so runners can be
seen approaching. With older
children, use colour-coded
beanbags to represent different
potatoes (red for hot, yellow
for warm, green for cool), so
that receivers have to decide
whether they must run, jog or
walk to pass on their potato.

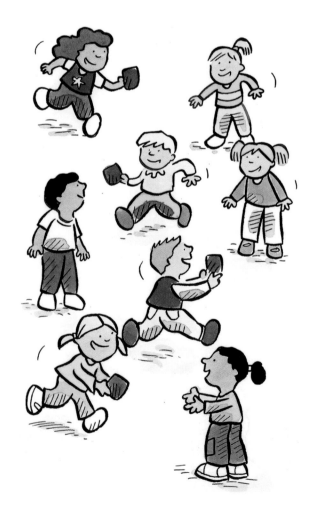

Home partnership

Encourage parents and carers
to play similar games with
their children, such as 'Tag'
or 'Lose your shadow', to
develop their dodging skills.

Theme links
My body
Opposites
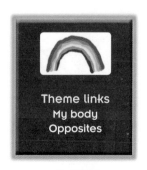

Further ideas

♦ Develop the children's
gentleness of touch by
playing the game using blown
eggs instead of beanbags or
small balls.
♦ Play the same game
outside on a hot, sunny day
using ice cubes.

Squiggles and swirls

Stepping Stone
Further explore an experience using a range of senses.

Early Learning Goal
Respond in a variety of ways to what they see, hear, smell, touch and feel.

Group size
Up to eight children.

What you need
Sealable transparent plastic bags; liquid paints; paper; sharp scissors (adult use); insulating tape.

What to do
Give each child a bag and invite them to choose three or four colours of paint. Squeeze a few centimetres of each colour into the children's bags and help them to completely seal them, excluding as much air as possible.

Encourage each child to gently press on the blobs of paint to disperse them and move them around inside the bag. Talk about what it feels like as the paint is manipulated. Ask the children to watch the colours as they begin to merge and mingle. Suggest that they close their eyes and squeeze the paint around, before opening their eyes again to see what has happened.

Invite each child to experiment by pressing their palm firmly down on the bag to move the paint, or pressing hard with their fingertips in a trail of distinct, separate movements, or even picking up the bag and squeezing, tipping or twisting it to create different effects. Periodically check the seams of the bag for splits, to avoid leakage.

Because the paint is sealed in, it will remain workable for a long time and so can be returned to as often as the child desires. To keep a particularly pleasing pattern, carefully cut around three sides of the bag, open it flat and take a print by gently pressing a sheet of paper on the paint.

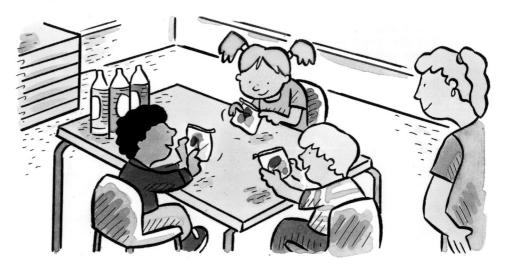

Support and extension
Seal the edges of the bags with insulating tape to make them stronger for very young children. Encourage older children to work with both hands to produce symmetrical patterns.

Home partnership
Parents will probably be willing to try this activity at home, since it is far less messy than the usual finger-painting activities, so suggest that they experiment by adding glitter or sugar to the bag.

Further ideas
♦ Provide opportunities for the children to make their own special, different-textured finger-paints by mixing flour, cornflour, glue or rice with paints.
♦ Give a different feel to tipping and pouring activities by using lentils or linseed instead of water or dry sand.

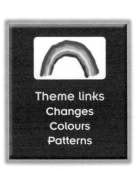

Theme links
Changes
Colours
Patterns

Foundation
Themes
Senses

Oooh, that tickles!

Stepping Stone
Show curiosity, observe and manipulate objects.

Early Learning Goal
Investigate objects and materials by using all of their senses as appropriate.

Group size
Up to six children.

What you need
A box containing a variety of objects with different textures and feels (preferably one of each for each child), for example, fluffy pompoms, feathers, pumice stones, loofahs, balls of soft dough, scrubbing brushes and cooked spaghetti; notepad and pen, or tape recorder (adult use).

What to do

Introduce the first object to the group and talk about what it is, where it came from and what it is used for. Explain to the children that you would like to know how the object feels to them: is it tickly, rough, cold or bumpy?

Give each child an object to handle and encourage them to use their own words to describe its feel. As the children investigate, tape their words or jot them down on the notepad for later reference.

Encourage each child to touch the object against their cheek, or the more sensitive inner part of their arm, and to say how it feels. Suggest that they close their eyes to help them to concentrate on the feel, rather than the look, of the object. Repeat the activity, using a different object each time.

Finally, gather the group together to listen to the tape, or to hear some of the key words that you have jotted down, and see if they can guess which objects the speaker was referring to.

Support and extension

Be ready with prompts to support and develop the vocabulary of very young children, who may find it difficult to express themselves clearly. Encourage older children to discuss similarities as well as differences in the feel of various objects. A sponge and a flannel, for example, are both soft, but a sponge is more squashy, and a feather is similar to a paintbrush, as part of it is hard and part is soft.

Home partnership

Ask parents and carers to help their children to develop their sense of touch by playing blindfold games, where an object is identified by touch alone.

Further ideas

♦ Challenge the children to complete simple tasks, such as doing up buttons or buckling a shoe, by touch alone.
♦ Create a wall collage of your local area using appropriate textures, such as sandpaper houses with transparent plastic windows, woodchip trees, thick black painted roads and textile people.

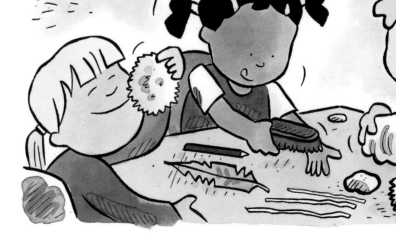

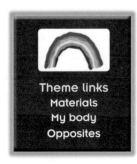

Theme links
Materials
My body
Opposites

Foundation Themes
Senses

I can write

Group size
Up to four children.

What you need
Four shallow trays; shaving foam; dry sand; custard powder; water; towel; lentils; strong feathers, short sticks or blunt pencils; pens and paper (adult use).

Preparation
Put a layer of dry sand in the first tray, lentils in the second, a thick paste of custard powder and water in the third and a layer of shaving foam in the fourth.

What to do
Invite the children to select a tray and investigate its contents by making marks and trails with their fingers. After a few minutes, let them wash and dry their hands if necessary, then encourage them to swap with a friend and try a different tray.

Talk to the children about how the different substances feel and react when drawn or written in. Ask them if one substance is better at retaining a trail than the other. Can anyone say why? Can the children draw a large circle in their tray before the substance goes back into place and erases the outline?

Introduce the implements and let the children experiment with mark-making, rotating the trays after a short while, until they have all experienced all the substances. Ask if any of the children prefer a particular tray. Can they say why? Do they prefer using their fingers or the sticks?

Challenge the children to each draw a smiley face, or write their initial or whole name in their tray.

Close the activity with a few minutes of free explorative play, allowing the children to take turns at various trays at will.

Support and extension
Write single letter shapes on paper for very young children to copy. Encourage older children to try to write a friend's name, instead of their own.

Home partnership
Encourage parents and carers to let their children practise mark-making activities at home, for example, using a clean brush and water, 'painting' shapes and letters on an outside fence or paving area.

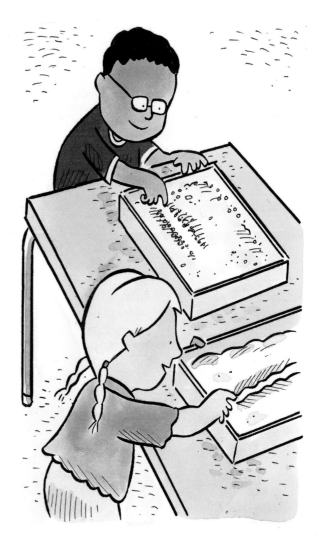

Further ideas
♦ Write the children's names on pieces of card and invite them to make textured name cards by tracing over the letters with glue and sprinkling them with sand, lentils or glitter.
♦ Mix white glue with shaving foam and use this thickly to write the children's names on black paper. When dry, the letters will be soft and puffy.

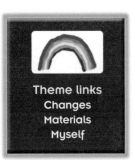

Theme links
Changes
Materials
Myself

Foundation Themes
Senses

Count the buttons

Stepping Stone
Count up to three or four objects by saying one number name for each item.

Group size
Up to four children.

What you need
Large wooden cube; buttons; strong glue; number line marked 1 to 10 for each child; 40 counters; blindfold.

Preparation
Make a dice by gluing one, two, three or four buttons on each face of the cube. (Use four only once, otherwise the game will be over too quickly.)

What to do
Give each child a number line and place the counters in the centre of the playing area. Explain to the children that they are going to play a game to try to fill the line with counters.

Count together along the line as you point to the numerals and agree that there are ten places to be filled. Show the children the dice and count together the different amounts of buttons on each face.

Explain that that was too easy, so the game has something else added to make it more difficult. Show the children the blindfold and invite them to guess how it might be used. Agree that the counting of the buttons on the dice has to be done by touch alone and ask for a volunteer to take the first turn.

Play the game by taking turns to wear the blindfold, count the buttons on the top face of the dice and collect the correct amount of counters from the central heap. Then uncover the eyes and place the counters in the spaces on the number line, one in each space. The game ends when everyone has filled their line with counters and checked to make sure that there are ten.

Early Learning Goal
Count reliably up to 10 everyday objects.

Support and extension
For very young children, who may be scared of wearing a blindfold, shield their view with a piece of fabric instead. Encourage older children to say which number they think they will move to on their number line, *before* they actually place their counters.

Home partnership
Invite parents and carers in to play simple board games, such as 'Snakes and ladders', with their children.

Further ideas
♦ Copy the photocopiable sheet 'Roll and count' on page 91 on to card and cut it out to make separate game cards, then use as above. The aim is to roll the dice, feel and count the dots, and stack that amount of counters on the appropriate square. The winner is the one that fills their card correctly first.
♦ Play 'Follow-my-leader fives' by following the person at the front of the line while they make five identical movements. The second in line then taps the leader on the shoulder, sends them to the back and takes over as leader.

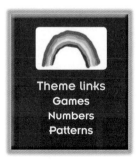

Theme links
Games
Numbers
Patterns

Foundation Themes
Senses

Tactile tunnels

Group size
Two to three children.

What you need
Cardboard tubes; strong glue; small pieces of different textured materials, such as sandpaper, corduroy, velvet, fur and so on (ten in all); scissors.

Preparation
Cut the tubes into 5cm or 6cm lengths and cut open one side to make tunnels. Glue a small piece of material on the 'ceiling' of each tunnel, making ten different pairs of identical textures.

What to do
Explain that you are going to play a game that relies on your hands, rather than your eyes, to tell you when two things are the same. Invite the children to put their fingers carefully under a tunnel to find out what the 'ceiling' feels like. Suggest that they close their eyes to help them to concentrate and to lessen the temptation to peek. Then encourage them to describe what they feel and allow them several minutes, so that they can explore a variety of tunnels.

Then arrange the tunnels into four neat rows of five columns. Demonstrate how to play, by feeling under a tunnel and describing its ceiling ('It's furry'), then feeling another and describing that one ('Oh, this one is bumpy'). Ask the children to try to remember what you said about each tunnel.

Invite a volunteer to play next, feeling under one tunnel, then another, and describing the textures. If someone thinks that they have discovered two identical textures, turn them over to check by looking.

If the player is correct, they win the tunnels, which are removed from the playing grid, and the player has another turn. If the player is not correct, the tunnels are returned to their original position and play passes to the next person. The game continues until there are no more tunnels on the grid. The winner is the one with the most tunnels.

Support and extension
Use only five pairs of tunnels for very young children, gradually building up the amount as they become more proficient. Let older children make the tunnels themselves, helping them if necessary.

Home partnership
Explain the game to parents and carers and suggest that they might like to make a set of tunnels to play with at home.

Further ideas
♦ Make a set of 'Touch snap' cards by sticking different textures on to squares of card, making sure that there are ten textures and 40 cards. When two identical cards are upturned, the player must shout an appropriately descriptive word, such as, 'furry', 'rough' or 'smooth', in order to win them.
♦ Read the rhyme 'How does it feel?' on the photocopiable sheet on page 84 and sing the song 'Touch' on the photocopiable sheet on page 87 with the children.

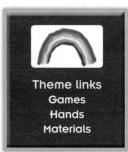

Theme links
Games
Hands
Materials

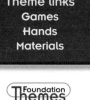
Foundation
Themes
Senses

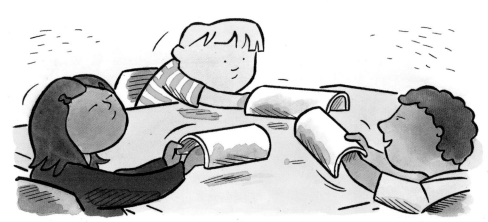

Feel the shape

Early Learning Goal
Move with control and co-ordination.

Group size
Six to eight children.

What you need
A familiar tray puzzle of four to six pieces, or a posting box; blindfold or piece of fabric.

What to do

Spend some time letting the children do the puzzle to ensure that they find it easy. Then suggest that it might not be quite so easy if they could not see what they were doing. How would they know which piece fitted where? (By feeling its shape.)

Introduce the blindfold and ask for a volunteer to take the first turn. Fit the blindfold and invite the child to remove the puzzle pieces from the tray and then put them back in again. Be ready to push pieces back within the child's reach or pick them up if they fall on the floor.

Give verbal support and encouragement as the child works, and be ready to offer practical strategies if they begin to lose interest or become frustrated. Say, for example, 'Try holding the tray with one hand and I'll pass a piece of puzzle into your other hand, to see if that helps'. If a child does give up, congratulate them on any success that they have had so far and invite them to finish the puzzle without the blindfold.

If a child seems uncomfortable using the blindfold, shield their vision with a piece of fabric instead. Once everyone has had a turn, tell the children that you will leave the blindfold and puzzle out for them to play with again, with a friend if they want to.

Support and extension

Support younger children by giving them verbal clues, such as, 'It's in the right place, now turn it around slowly,' or, 'Can you feel the bumpy bit to fit in the hole?'. Challenge older children further by setting a time limit or providing them with a bigger puzzle.

Home partnership

Suggest that the children challenge their parents and carers to complete one of their puzzles by touch alone.

Further ideas

♦ Arrange drawing pins into letter or number shapes by pushing them into a piece of softwood, and let the children feel the protruding heads and try to guess what the numbers are without looking.

♦ Invite the children to thread beads or pile cubes into a tower without looking.

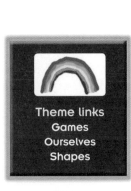

Theme links
Games
Ourselves
Shapes

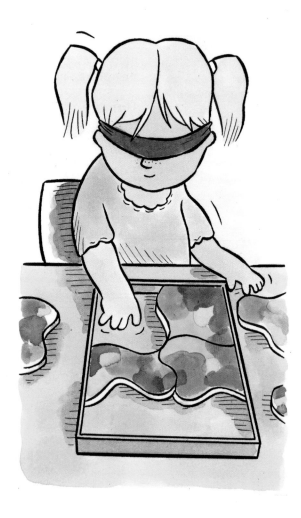

Foundation
Themes
Senses

Here's one!

Stepping Stone
Select a particular named shape.

Early Learning Goal
Use language such as 'circle' or 'bigger' to describe the shape and size of solids and flat shapes.

Group size
Up to four children.

What you need
Large shallow tray; cornflour; water; flat plastic shapes.

Preparation
Mix the cornflour with water to make a thick paste, and note how many of each shape are in the set for later reference.

What to do
Look at the shapes together and practise naming and identifying each one. Ensure that each child is familiar with at least some of the properties of each shape.

Spread the shapes out and ask the children to take it in turns to select a particular shape. Congratulate them on how clever they are, then invite them to take part in a messy challenge.

Put the shapes into the shallow tray and cover them with the cornflour mixture. Ask for a volunteer to find a triangle by feeling in the paste. Remind them to feel the outline of the shape carefully to make sure that it is a triangle before picking it up.

If they are correct, the shape is removed from the tray; if not, it goes back in. Continue to take turns to select shapes until the whole set has been collected.

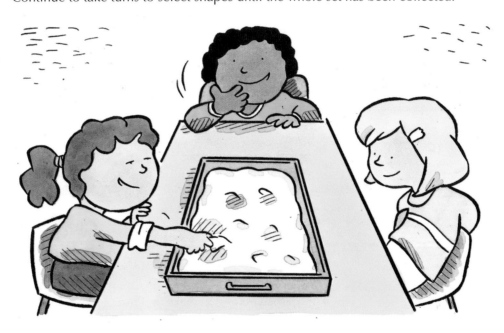

Support and extension
Some very young children may be wary of putting their hands into the mixture, so give them a small, individual tray of paste to explore in their own time before expecting them to take part in the more structured activity. Challenge older children to find a shape with particular properties, rather than naming it – for example, 'Find a shape that is big and has no corners'. Ask them to name it once they have found it.

Home partnership
Encourage parents and carers to play 'Feel and guess' games with familiar objects at home, by asking their children to put their hands behind their back and giving them an object to handle and name.

Further ideas
♦ Repeat the activity using 3-D shapes hidden among shredded paper, or familiar objects buried in peat.
♦ Make a set of textured shapes, hide them indoors or outdoors, and challenge the children to find, for example, a soft triangle, a rough square or a bumpy circle.

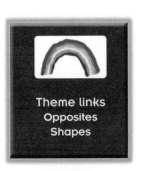

Theme links
Opposites
Shapes

Stir, mix, stretch and pull

Early Learning Goal
Explore colour, texture, shape, form and space in two or three dimensions.

Group size
Up to four children.

What you need
A bowl for each child; flour; salt; water; aprons; cups; spoons; rice; sand; glitter; shredded Cellophane; sawdust; small, sealable plastic bags.

What to do
Help each child to put on an apron and give them a bowl. Explain that they are going to invent their own play dough using some of the things on the table. Invite them to tip two cupfuls of flour and one cupful of salt into their bowl and stir it around with their hands. Then, let them select one more dry ingredient to spoon into their bowl, to give their dough an interesting feel, and mix it in well.

Ask the children what they think they need next to hold the mixture together and make it into dough. (Water.) Suggest that they stir in half a cupful of water at first and add extra when necessary, allowing them to decide how much water they need (but be prepared with extra flour if things become a little too sticky!). Encourage the children to talk about their dough and what it feels like, asking if it is dry, stretchy, lumpy, gritty or crumbly.

Once their dough is well mixed, invite the children to manipulate it using their hands, flattening it, rolling it, breaking it into pieces and moulding it into shapes, as they wish. Suggest that they might like to share some of their dough with the others, so that they can compare the different types and see which they like the most.

This is an experiential activity and works best if the children are able to pursue it for as long as their interest is maintained. Sealed in a plastic bag and stored in a refrigerator, the dough should stay malleable for several days, allowing the children to use it as and when desired.

Support and extension
Very young children may need help to mix the water into the flour. Encourage older children to be really inventive with their descriptive vocabulary.

Home partnership
Suggest that the children each make a small object, such as a butterfly, snake or snail, leave it to dry, paint it and then take it home to keep.

Further ideas
♦ Help the children to make and use papier mâché.
♦ Provide opportunities for the children to make mud pies in a controlled environment, using soil, spoons, twigs, leaves and stones.

Theme links
Changes
Materials

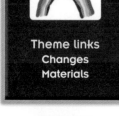

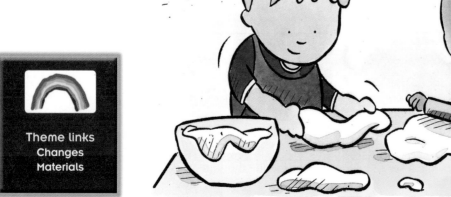

Chapter 3

Hearing

Use the world of sound to stimulate the children's mathematical development, foster an interest in the world about them, motivate them to speak clearly and encourage them to think of others as well as themselves, as they take part in the variety of activities contained within this chapter.

Group size
Whole group.

What you need
Percussion instrument; space to move freely.

Preparation
Spend a few minutes beating out some different rhythms for the group to listen to and differentiate between.

Stand up, shake, sit

What to do
Tell the children that the rhythms that you are playing make you feel as though you want to move. Play a slow, steady rhythm and say that it sounds like 'hopping' music.

Ask the children to listen to it again and invite them to hop along to the beat. Suggest that if one leg gets tired they can hop on the other foot instead. Play the same rhythm at various speeds and encourage the children to keep time with their hopping.

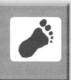

Stepping Stone
Respond to rhythm, music and story by means of gesture and movement.

Early Learning Goal
Move with confidence, imagination and in safety.

After a few minutes, sit the group down and play a different rhythm, reminding the children to listen carefully and agreeing on a suitable movement, before inviting them to join in. Repeat the exercise three or four times, using a different rhythm each time. Use some short sequences too, to signify, for example, shaking, spinning or freezing.

Finally, gather the group together to listen once more to each rhythm and encourage the children to tell you how they moved to it. Finish the session by suggesting a game, where you play a random selection of the rhythms and the children try to do the associated movements without being reminded.

Support and extension
Help younger children to differentiate between the rhythms by using a different instrument for each one. Encourage older children to create their own individual movements to suit each rhythm, rather than imposing the same movements on the whole group.

Home partnership
Encourage each child to bring in a favourite music tape or CD from home, and set aside approximately ten minutes for the children to listen and move freely to it.

Further ideas
♦ Beat out a rhythm while the children use felt-tipped pens or paints to make an associated pattern on large sheets of paper.
♦ Take a portable music centre outside and give the children lengths of ribbon to whirl and swirl as they dance along to various types of music.

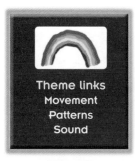

Theme links
Movement
Patterns
Sound

Foundation
Themes
Senses

Crash, twang, boom!

Group size
Up to six children.

What you need
A selection of drums, cymbals, gongs, beaters, elastic bands and strong boxes of various shapes and sizes (some with holes in and some without); small pieces of wood or prisms of card to use as bridges and stretchers.

What to do

Gather the group together and talk about the selection of equipment and what it might be for. Invite one child to select an item and try to make a sound with it. Then ask them to pass it to a friend and see if they can make a different sound with the same item.

Talk about the different sounds and the way that they were made. Repeat this a few times until all the children have had at least one turn to create a sound. Invite the group to explore all the items, experimenting with them to see what sounds they can produce.

Work alongside the children, encouraging them to use the elastic bands on different boxes and the wood to stretch them. Ask them to listen carefully to notice how the sounds, produced from the same elastic band, differ when it is plucked, struck or scraped. Let them investigate the difference that a hole makes to the sound produced from a box.

Finally, ask each child to think about which is their favourite sound from all those that they have produced. Suggest that they form a band and each play their sound to accompany you all as you sing a favourite nursery rhyme or song.

Support and extension

Help very young children to distinguish different sounds by using the words 'high' and 'low' appropriately, and encouraging them to do the same. Challenge older children to produce a high, a medium and a low note from the same elastic band.

Home partnership

Ask the children to bring in recyclable materials from home, make a variety of instruments or sound-makers and decorate them attractively.

Further ideas

♦ Set up a working display of commercial and home-produced instruments (see 'Changing sounds' on page 80).
♦ Invite in a local musician to demonstrate the range of sounds that can be produced from one instrument.

Theme links
Changes
Opposites
Sound

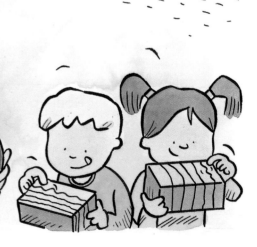

Foundation
Themes
Senses

Very carefully

Group size
12 to 15 children.

What you need
Rainstick; tambourine; bells.

What to do
Split the group into two and sit them facing one another approximately 5m apart. Show the children the rainstick and demonstrate how it works. Ask them to listen to the sound slowly fading away, then move the stick slightly, so that it makes sound again.

Early Learning Goal
Show awareness of space, of themselves and of others.

Challenge the children to pass the stick back and forth to each other without letting it make a noise. Start the activity off yourself by carefully carrying the stick to the first child. If it makes a sound, even when you are handing it to the child, stop and go back to your starting-point.

Continue in this way until the last child has brought the stick back to you. Remind the waiting children to listen carefully all the time in case the stick makes a sound. Repeat the activity using the tambourine and finally the bells.

Talk about which instrument the children had most success with and discuss why that might be. Congratulate the children on their careful handling of the items and leave these accessible for them to use at their leisure.

Support and extension
If very young children find it too difficult to carry the stick while moving, play the game in a circle. Challenge older children by imposing restrictions, such as using only one hand, or hopping or crawling with the stick.

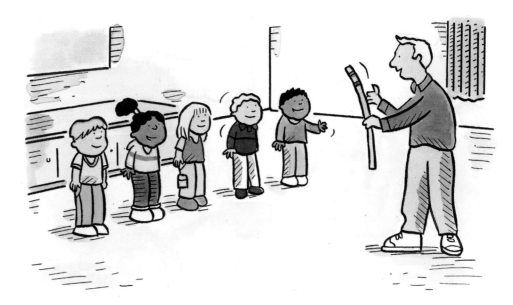

Home partnership
Explain to parents and carers what you have been doing and ask them to help their children to practise moving carefully by setting them challenges, such as climbing into the bath water or walking on a gravel path without making a sound.

Further ideas
♦ Give the children further challenges, such as carrying a ball on a tray over a set course, and encourage them to think of challenges for themselves and one another.
♦ Set up an area with closely packed cones or markers and encourage the children to weave in and out without touching them, gradually increasing the difficulty level by going faster, carrying something or dribbling a ball.

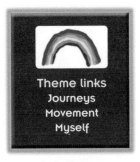

Theme links
Journeys
Movement
Myself

Foundation
Themes
Senses

How many steps?

Group size
Eight children.

What you need
The photocopiable sheet 'How far does it travel?' on page 92; large outdoor space; two adults; triangle; drum; bell; recorder; four coloured cones or markers, each labelled with the name of one of the instruments; writing materials; clipboards.

Preparation
Make a copy of the photocopiable sheet for each child.

What to do
Gather the children together and listen to the sound of each instrument in turn. Talk about the comparative loudness of the tones and ask the children to guess which one they think might make the most noise. Suggest that you check if anyone is right by measuring how far away the sound can be heard.

Give four children a different coloured marker each and assign them to one adult, then give the other four an instrument each and ask them to stay with the remaining adult. Explain that the children with the instruments are going to stay where they are, but those with the markers will be walking further and further away.

Decide upon a starting instrument and ask the child to keep playing it while the marker group walks away. When the marker group can no longer hear the sound, they must stop and place the relevant marker on the spot. Repeat this with each instrument in turn.

Call the whole group back to the starting-point and discuss the findings of your experiment. Finally, count together how many adult paces each sound travelled and help each child to record the results on their copy of the photocopiable sheet.

Support and extension
With very young children, use just one activity sheet for the whole group rather than completing individual sheets. Encourage older children to measure the distances using a trundle wheel or tape measure.

Home partnership
Send home the completed activity sheets and encourage the children to explain their experiment to their families.

Further ideas
♦ Construct a dark-room and give the children torches and reflective surfaces for them to investigate freely.
♦ Provide a selection of magnets (both rigid and pliable) and a variety of magnetic and non-magnetic materials for the children to explore and discuss.

Theme links
Measuring
Sound

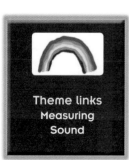

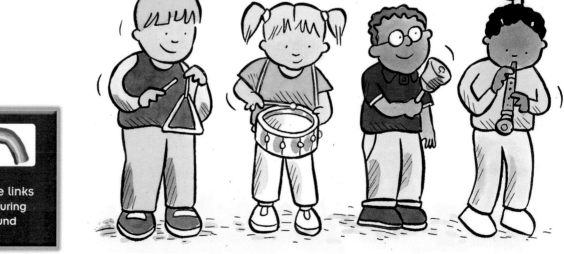

Left a bit, stop!

Early Learning Goal
Consider the consequences of their words and actions for themselves and others.

Group size
Four to six children.

What you need
Simple obstacle course: blindfolds.

What to do
Look at the obstacle course together and explain that the idea is to complete it by going around, under or over all the objects without touching them. Invite all the children to try the course and exclaim that it is obviously much too easy, so perhaps they could do it with their eyes closed. Let volunteers try the course blindfolded, but declare it too difficult and suggest that it might be easier if they helped each other.

Ask for another volunteer to wear the blindfold. Stand behind them and instruct them to move forward, step over or move to the left, as appropriate, to enable them to complete the course successfully. Discuss what you have done, stressing the importance of giving clear, correct instructions that the partner can understand. Talk about what might happen if wrong instructions are given.

Next, invite the children to find partners and take turns to wear the blindfold or give instructions. Ask the instructors to walk behind their partners and, if necessary, to touch them gently on an arm to signify left or right. Remind blindfolded children to listen very carefully the whole time and to do exactly what their partner says.

As the children work, walk among them, praising any clear, precise instructions and any careful listening that you notice.

Finish the session by gathering the group together and talking about the activity, reinforcing the idea that tasks can often be made easier if we help one another.

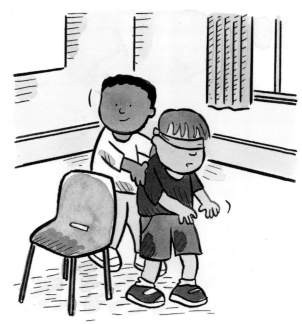

Support and extension
Pair very young children with an adult until they are confident enough to partner another child. Encourage older children to use precise directional language, including the words 'left' and 'right'.

Home partnership
Explain the game to parents and carers and ask them to practise it at home with their children.

Further ideas
♦ Set fun challenges to encourage the children to work in pairs, such as practising three-legged walking, or cutting up bread, with a friend, using a knife and fork.
♦ Play 'Message relays' by giving pairs of children messages to relay to each other, for example, 'Clap hands', or 'Jump up and down'. Award a point for each action performed correctly.

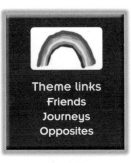

Theme links
Friends
Journeys
Opposites

Foundation **Themes**
Senses

Noisy or quiet?

Stepping Stone
Sort objects by one function.

Early Learning Goal
Ask questions about why things happen and how things work.

What you need
Group size
Up to four children.

What you need
A large selection of everyday objects, including a feather, a paper tissue and other soft, light items.

Preparation
This is primarily a thinking exercise to develop the children's logical thought processes, so there are no right or wrong answers – merely interesting ideas!

What to do
Look at all the objects together, inviting the children to identify and give a brief description of each one. Ask them to each select an item that can make a noise and to demonstrate that noise while the rest of the group listens.

Then, challenge each child to select an item that *cannot* make a sound. Invite them to test their theory by trying to make a sound with their chosen object. Suggest that if they do produce a sound they put that object back, but if they do not, they invite a friend to try before replacing the item.

Continually challenge the children by thinking aloud, for example, 'I wonder if the teddy could still make a noise if he wasn't allowed to touch anything except someone's hands?'.

Finally, leave the children with this thought: 'I wonder if the objects could make a sound if they were not touched at all?'. Leave them to investigate further in their own time if they wish.

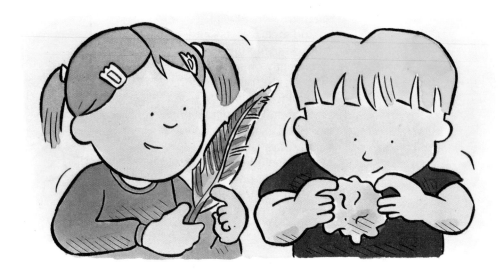

Support and extension
For very young children, work with only one or two children, to ensure optimum participation and concentration. Encourage older children to sort the objects according to their ability to produce a sound, with those producing little or no sound at one end and those that produce many sounds at the other.

Home partnership
Read the rhyme 'Peace and quiet' on page 84 to the children and encourage them to listen for loud sounds and quiet sounds in and around their own homes.

Further ideas
♦ Stock the water tray with a wide variety of containers that have holes, for example, pierced yoghurt pots and plastic tubes, strainers, sieves, sealed but pierced plastic bottles and so on, and encourage the children to discuss their behaviour in water.
♦ Investigate cubic bubbles and bubbles within bubbles by adding plastic straws and connectors to a deep tank of bubble liquid.
♦ Sing the song 'Listen very carefully' on the photocopiable sheet on page 87 with the children, carrying out the actions as instructed.

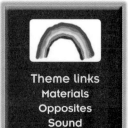

Theme links
Materials
Opposites
Sound

Foundation
Themes
Senses

One, two, three

Early Learning Goal
Count reliably up to 10 everyday objects.

Group size
Whole group.

What you need
A metronome or adjustable ticking pendulum.

What to do
Introduce the metronome to the group, explain what it is used for and demonstrate how it works. Suggest that it might be useful for practising counting and set it at a steady pace. Encourage the children to all close their eyes, listen carefully and join in as you count to the beat from one to ten. Then ask them to open their eyes.

Repeat the activity, this time using very quiet voices and opening eyes on the count of ten. Repeat it again, counting silently and asking the children to open their eyes when they have counted ten ticks. Develop the exercise further by stopping the metronome after a number of ticks and inviting the group to tell you how many ticks they have counted.

Once the children are familiar with the activity, adjust the metronome to practise counting at different speeds, more slowly as well as more quickly. Invite a confident child to adjust the instrument and count aloud in front of the group, while the others listen carefully. If anyone hears a mistake, they must shoot up their hand and say so. If their challenge is valid, they can take a turn to adjust the metronome, but if not, the first child takes another turn before choosing a successor.

Finish the activity by counting, as a whole group, at a steady pace, to 20 or more.

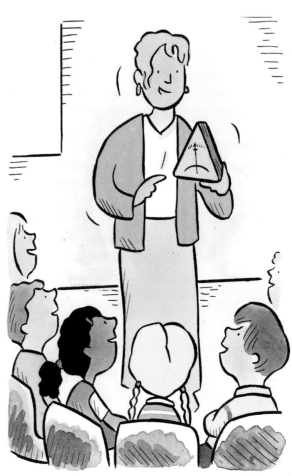

Support and extension
Younger children may need to keep their eyes open at first and count only to five. Challenge older children to count backwards, in twos, rapidly or beyond ten.

Theme links
Clocks
Rhythm and rhymes
Sound

Home partnership
Encourage the children to count sounds at home, including the ticks of a clock or timer, the rings of a telephone or knocks on a door.

Further ideas
♦ Use percussion instruments behind a screen to play more counting and listening games with the children.
♦ Play marching, hopping or jumping games, using a drum to regulate the beat as the children count their steps.

Foundation Themes
Senses

Tricky counting

What to do

Take your first set of objects and invite the group to count along as you place them, one by one, on the first surface. Then ask the children to watch and listen carefully while you count the objects again.

Tell the children to be ready to put up their hands to tell you if you make a mistake, because you might not be so clever at counting as they are. Count the objects as you move them to the second surface, one by one, making a mistake at some point to see if the children notice.

If they do, ask them what you should have said instead and continue counting from there. If they do not, repeat the activity and emphasise the mistake as you make it. Repeat this activity with different sets of objects, varying the difficulty by counting at different speeds.

Continue for as long as the children are interested and involved, making different types of error, pretending to move an object while continuing to count, or picking up two objects at once, so that the children have to use both sight and hearing to help them. Practise this activity regularly, increasing the difficulty level each time.

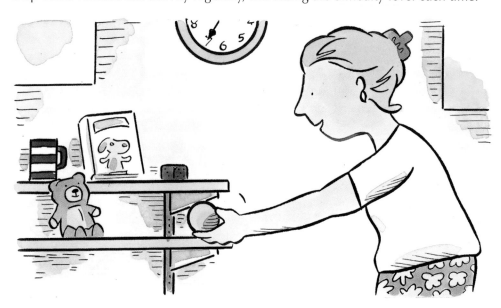

Support and extension

Use only five or six objects with very young children and, after a mistake has been spotted, re-count the moved objects to help the children to know which number will be next in the sequence. For older children, use more objects and try counting backwards on to the first surface or counting in multiples of two or three.

Home partnership

Set a simple counting problem for the children to solve at home, such as how many steps lead upstairs, or how many ears there are in their house.

Further ideas

♦ Print out the words to favourite counting rhymes on large sheets of paper and invite the children to illustrate them to make posters.
♦ Read the story of *The Six Foolish Fishermen* by Benjamin Elkin (Scholastic – out of print, try libraries) and talk about the mistake that they made.

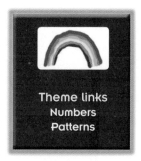

Theme links
Numbers
Patterns

Found it!

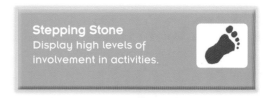

Stepping Stone
Display high levels of involvement in activities.

Early Learning Goal
Continue to be interested, excited and motivated to learn.

Group size
Six to eight children.

What you need
A timer or alarm clock with a loud tick; two cardboard boxes.

What to do
Encourage the children to be as quiet and still as possible while you listen to the timer together. Tell them that you are going to put the timer in a box and that they have to try to guess which box by listening very carefully for the tick.

Turn your back, so that the children cannot see the two boxes as you hold them in front of you and place the timer in one of them. Face the children again and hold one box in each hand out to the sides at arm's length.

Encourage the children to listen carefully and to put up their hands to tell you where the timer is. Practise this a few times to familiarise the children with the idea. Then ask them to close their eyes while you walk around the room and secretly hide the timer somewhere.

Invite the children to open their eyes and creep around listening carefully until they locate the timer. Once they can do this, set the timer to one minute, hide it in a less obvious place and challenge them to find it before it rings.

Support and extension
With younger children, this game will need to be played in a very quiet area to help them to concentrate on listening. Older children will be able to take turns to set and hide the timer for one another.

Home partnership
Ask parents and carers to challenge their children to see what they can do in one minute, for example, how many times they can run to the gate and back, how many smiley faces they can draw and so on.

Further ideas
♦ Enliven 'Hide-and-seek' games by giving the hiding children bells to wear around their ankles, so that the seeker will hear them when they move.
♦ Play 'Blind man's buff' to see if the children can recognise one another by the sound of their voices.

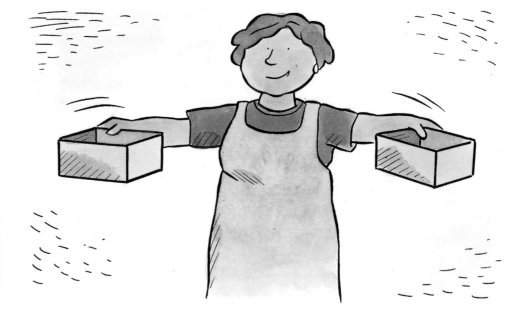

Theme links
Games
Sound
Time

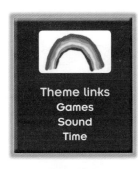

I know a little girl

Group size
Up to ten children.

What you need
One set of lower-case and two sets of upper-case letters or letter cards.

Preparation
The children will need to have had some experience of listening carefully before they are able to achieve success in this activity.

What to do
Tell the children that you have in your mind one particular child out of the group and that you would like them to guess who it is, after being given just one clue. Remind them to put up their hands, rather than calling out, when they think that they know who it is.

Next, say, for example, 'I know a little girl... and her name begins with... "cuh"'. If no one comes up with the correct answer, say the initial sound again, but continue a little further into sounding out the name. Carry on in this way until the name is finally guessed.

Invite the named child to come to the front and find the initial letter of her name from the set of capitals and show it to the group, while you all say its sound: '"Cuh" – "cuh" for "Catherine"'.

Repeat the activity until each child has had a turn to identify and find the initial sound and letter of their name. Finish the activity by pointing at each child in turn as you say their initial sound and name, for example, '"Duh" – "duh" for "Dipak"; "Ssss" – "ssss" for "Sasha"'. Encourage the children to join in too.

Support and extension
Help very young children to each find their initial letter by giving them one to match it with. Challenge older children to find the lower-case counterpart of their name's initial capital letter.

Home partnership
Encourage parents and carers to help their children to identify and write the initial letter of everyone in their household and bring the list in to share with the group.

Further ideas
♦ Hide a familiar object in a box, hold up its initial letter (lower case), say its sound and ask the children to guess what it might be.
♦ Play 'I hear with my little ear' both indoors and outdoors.

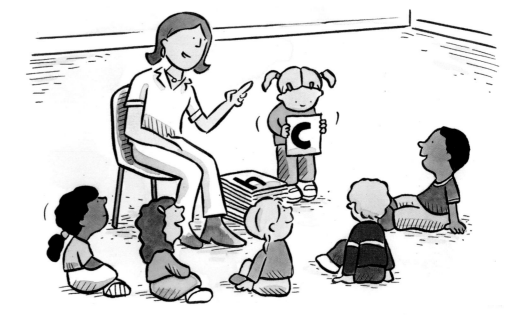

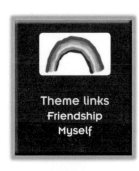

Theme links
Friendship
Myself

It's stopped!

Early Learning Goal
Recognise and explore how sounds can be changed, sing simple songs from memory, recognise repeated sounds and sound patterns and match movements to music.

Group size
Whole group.

What you need
Handbell; triangle; cymbal; drum; beaters; small selection of other or similar musical instruments.

What to do

Look at the instruments together and ensure that the children are familiar with the names. Encourage them to close their eyes and listen carefully while you strike the drum. Ask if they think that it was a long sound or a short one. Strike it again, so that they can check.

Invite the children to close their eyes again while you strike the second instrument, but this time they must keep their eyes closed until the sound has stopped. Was that sound longer or shorter than the first one?

Repeat with each instrument in turn, each time noticing how long the sound lasted. Then select one instrument and ask the children to watch and listen carefully. Strike the instrument and immediately hold or touch it to stop its sound. Ask the children to explain what happened.

Encourage volunteers to come forward and try the same experiment with each of the other instruments. At the end of the session, tell the group that you will leave out the instruments, along with several others, for them to experiment with on their own.

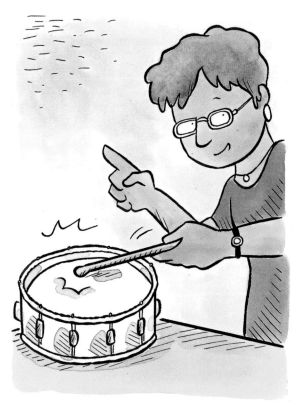

Support and extension

Younger children may find it hard to keep their eyes closed as long as necessary, so invite them to stand up while you strike the instrument, and sit down when they can no longer hear it. Encourage older children to measure the length of the sounds by regular counting or using a stopwatch, and record the results on a simple graph.

Home partnership

Invite in a musical parent or carer to play an instrument for the group to listen to. Talk about how long or short the notes that are played on it are.

Further ideas

♦ Alter 'Musical statues' by agreeing upon a different posture for each instrument, such as a star shape for the triangle, a crouch for the drum and so on. Let the children skip and dance freely until you strike an instrument, when they must adopt and hold the posture until the sound has faded away.

♦ Clap or stamp along to music, loudly at first and slowly becoming quieter as you gradually fade out the sound.

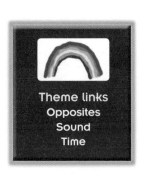

Theme links
Opposites
Sound
Time

Foundation
Themes
Senses

There's a little house...

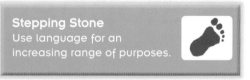

Early Learning Goal
Speak clearly and audibly with
confidence and control and
show awareness of the listener,
for example by their use of
conventions such as greetings,
'please' and 'thank you'.

Group size
Pairs of children.

What you need
Painting or drawing
equipment.

Preparation
Ensure that the
children have
had plenty of
free drawing
and painting
experience and are
confident to make
marks on paper.

What to do
Invite a child to select a friend that they would like to work with and tell them that they are going to be taking turns to draw or paint. Ask them to decide who is going to go first and give them the necessary equipment, but tell them that they must not start yet.

Explain that each child is not going to do their own picture, but their friend is going to tell them what to do instead. Invite the instructor to say what they would like in the picture and encourage the artist to draw it.

Say that the picture can be of real things or of things that do not exist, as long as the instructions are clear. As they work, ask questions to encourage the instructor to give precise and detailed instructions, for example, 'What colour is it?', 'Where do you want it to go?' and so on.

When the pictures are complete, encourage the children to look at them together and point out relevant features, for example, saying, 'Oh look, there's the yellow circle you asked for in the corner!'. Then invite them to swap roles and repeat the activity.

Support and extension
Pair very young children with an adult, so that they can simplify instructions accordingly and be able to draw a reasonable representation of whatever the child asks for, in order to avoid frustration. Extend the activity for older children, by screening them from each other and inviting them both to draw the picture and compare results.

Home partnership
Encourage parents and carers to play 'Simon says' at home, taking turns with their child to be 'Simon' and issue the instructions.

Further ideas
♦ Try the activity with construction equipment or recyclable modelling materials.
♦ Take pairs of children shopping and give them the opportunity to do all the talking necessary to complete the transaction.

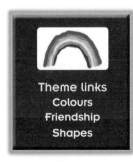
Theme links
Colours
Friendship
Shapes

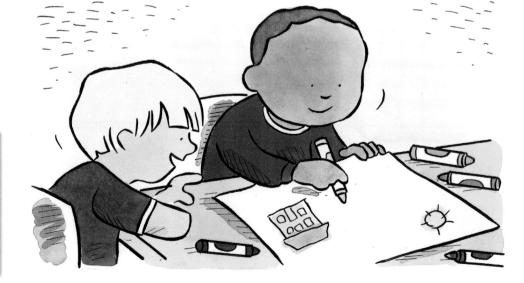

Chapter 4

Taste

Most children are interested in food, and the activities in this chapter will encourage them to try unfamiliar foods as well as to think and talk about some old favourites. The ideas will also encourage the children to explore shape and size, use everyday technology and develop their physical dexterity.

Is it this one?

Group size
Six children.

What you need
A selection of fruit (some familiar and some unusual), at least two pieces of each variety; food-preparation and serving equipment; labels; writing materials.

Preparation
Leave one piece of each fruit intact and display it for the group to see and handle. Prepare the rest of the fruit, placing each variety in a separate container and keeping it covered until required.

Check for any food allergies or dietary requirements.

What to do
Gather the group together to examine your selection of whole fruit. Talk about each fruit in turn, remarking upon its colour, size and texture. Discuss how it grows and where it comes from. Write out a name label to place by each fruit.

Invite the children to sit down and bring out the first tasting bowl, passing it around for each child to take a piece. Encourage the children to smell the fruit before tasting it. Help them to vocalise their feelings about the piece of fruit and ask them to suggest which whole fruit it matches.

Place the bowl beside the suggested whole fruit and bring out the next one. Continue in this way until the children have tasted all the pieces of fruit and matched each of the bowls with the whole fruit. Then take the first bowl and fruit and tell the children that you are going to see if their guess was correct by slicing open the whole fruit.

If the children were right, congratulate them and move on to the next fruit. If they were wrong, explain that one of the other pairs must be wrong too and give them a chance to put it right. Continue the process with the remaining fruit. Draw the activity to a close by asking the children to name each fruit in turn.

Stepping Stone
Have a positive approach to new experiences.

Early Learning Goal
Be confident to try new activities, initiate ideas and speak in a familiar group.

Support and extension
Cut the fruit into tiny pieces to encourage reluctant children to taste them all. Invite older children to both name each fruit and say a few words about it.

Home partnership
Ask parents and carers to bring in any unusual fruit that they see while out shopping, complete with a country-of-origin sticker if possible.

Further ideas
♦ Have a blind tasting of familiar foodstuffs.
♦ Show the photocopiable sheet 'Match the fruit' on page 93 to the children and encourage them to identify the pairs of fruit and to colour them as realistically as they can.

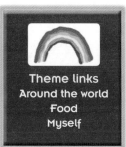

Theme links
Around the world
Food
Myself

Foundation Themes
Senses

Oops!

Stepping Stone
Engage in activities requiring hand–eye co-ordination.

Early Learning Goal
Handle tools, objects, construction and malleable materials safely and with increasing control.

Group size
Up to four children.

What you need
A pair of plastic chopsticks for each child; small bowls; rice; spaghetti; peas; beans; aprons; kitchen roll; elastic bands (optional).

Preparation
Prepare the foodstuffs and place a little of each into separate bowls.

Check for any food allergies or dietary requirements.

What to do

Look at the chopsticks together and talk about what they are and how they are used. If there is a child who is proficient in their use, ask them to demonstrate their technique.

Next, explain that you have some food prepared for the children, but they must use the chopsticks to pick it up. Give each child an apron, a pair of chopsticks and a bowl of food. Stand by with the kitchen roll to mop up any spills!

Encourage the children to persevere even if they keep dropping the food. Suggest that they hold their bowls close to their mouths, so that they do not have to carry the food for longer than necessary. If they are really struggling, wrap an elastic band around the end of their chopsticks to make them more controllable.

Give each child the opportunity to try each different foodstuff to see which they find easiest to manipulate. At the end of the session, talk about what you have been doing and encourage the children to say what they felt about the experience.

Support and extension

For very young children, provide simpler foods, such as crisps or small pieces of pizza, to begin with. Extend the activity for older children by giving them empty bowls and a serving dish to collect their food from.

Home partnership

Wash the chopsticks thoroughly and give a pair to each child to take home, so that they can continue practising, perhaps using pieces of bread.

Further ideas

♦ Play a relay game using chopsticks to transfer beads or small cubes from one place to another.
♦ Provide the children with a tray full of cooked, lightly oiled spaghetti, small dishes and a variety of spoons, forks, tongs and other serving implements, so that they can develop their dexterity.

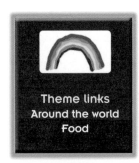

Theme links
Around the world
Food

Foundation Themes
Senses

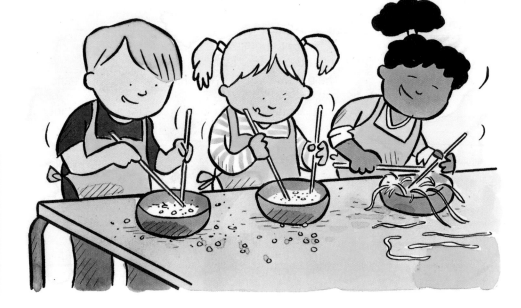

That one is the biggest!

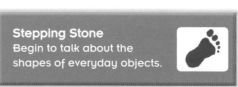

Stepping Stone
Begin to talk about the shapes of everyday objects.

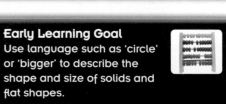

Early Learning Goal
Use language such as 'circle' or 'bigger' to describe the shape and size of solids and flat shapes.

Group size
Four children.

What you need
A selection of biscuits in various shapes and sizes; tray; cling film or small, sealable, transparent bags; paper plates.

Preparation
Wrap each individual biscuit securely in cling film, or enclose it in a sealed bag, and put the biscuits all together on the tray.

> Check for any food allergies or dietary requirements.

What to do
Look at the biscuits together and talk about their similarities and differences regarding shape and size. Explain to the children that the food is all jumbled and needs sorting out, but you are not quite sure how to do it. Give them the plates and ask them if they can do it for you. Observe them as they work, encouraging them to explain what they are doing and to use mathematical terms to describe the biscuits that they are sorting.

When they have completed the task to their satisfaction, ask them to explain why they have sorted them in that particular way. Then think of a different way of sorting them yourself, but stop before the task is complete and invite the children to finish for you.

Finally, spread out the plates and tell the children that they are allowed to each have a biscuit of their choice, but first they must describe it accurately so that you can select the right one for them. Let each child take a turn to describe their chosen biscuit. If you are able to select the one that they wanted, they can have it and, if not, put it back, move on to the next child and return to them later for another turn.

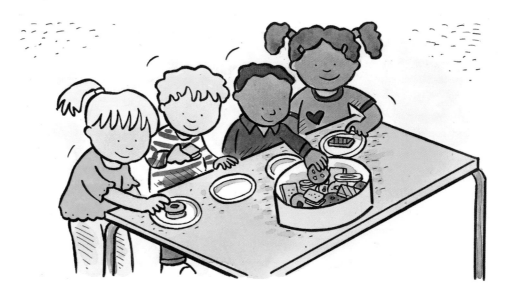

Support and extension
The biscuits will survive longer in very young hands if they are placed in sealed transparent containers, rather than bags or film. Invite older children to work in pairs, with the first child starting the sorting, without explaining their reasoning, and the second completing the task, trying to use the same criteria.

Home partnership
Encourage parents and carers to help their children to spot different shapes of items in the supermarket when they are shopping.

Further ideas
♦ Set up the home corner as a shop. Label shelves and packets with different shapes and invite 'shelf-stackers' to sort the items on to appropriate shelves.
♦ Display a selection of biscuits and challenge the children to replicate some of them, using coloured dough.

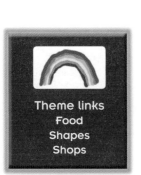

Theme links
Food
Shapes
Shops

Foundation Themes
Senses

Easter bonnets

Group size
Up to six children.

What you need
Cooking equipment; hot water; aprons; digestive biscuits; marshmallows; chocolate; tiny sugar shapes; sugar strands.

Preparation
Ensure that the cooking area and equipment are hygienically clean and the children's hands thoroughly washed. Make a sample bonnet biscuit yourself, following the instructions in 'What to do'.

Check for any food allergies or dietary requirements.

What to do

Help each child to put on an apron. Show the children the bonnet that you made earlier and explain that they are each going to make one of their own.

Introduce the ingredients and ask the children how they think they should proceed. Lead them to realise that the base biscuit must first be coated in chocolate, therefore the chocolate must be melted. So invite them to snap the chocolate into small pieces and place these in a bowl.

Place the bowl in hot water and let the children watch as you stir until the chocolate has melted. Remove the bowl from the water and invite each child to pour a spoonful of chocolate on to their biscuit and tip it around until the top is covered. Leave it to harden for a few minutes while you discuss what to do next.

Then give each child a fork and invite them to stab a marshmallow securely, dip it into the chocolate and place it in the centre of their biscuit.

Finally, decorate the bonnet with the sugar shapes and strands and leave to dry.

Support and extension

Use chocolate biscuits with very young children, rather than asking them to coat their own. If they are very carefully supervised, older children will be able to stir the melting chocolate for themselves.

Home partnership

Once the bonnets are dry, wrap them in cling film and let the children take them home, so that they can talk with their families about what they have been doing.

Further ideas

♦ Add a little liquid detergent to the water tray and provide a variety of whisks and beaters for the children to beat up a lather.
♦ Decorate plain biscuits with icing using a syringe or piping bag.

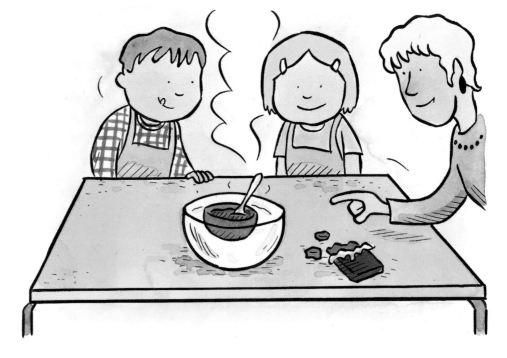

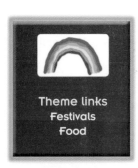

Theme links
Festivals
Food

Foundation
Themes
Senses

Finger-food buffet

Stepping Stone
Express needs and feelings in appropriate ways.

Early Learning Goal
Have a developing awareness of their own needs, views and feelings and be sensitive to the needs, views and feelings of others.

Group size
Groups of four children, then the whole group.

What you need
Hygienic food preparation area; serving equipment, including tables and cloths; wide selection of finger foods; blankets; weak squash.

Check for any food allergies or dietary requirements.

What to do
Gather four volunteers and help them to prepare some of the food and arrange it on serving plates. Encourage them to talk about the food that they are preparing and remind them not to start nibbling just yet! Cover the food until it is required.

Continue with new groups of four, until all the food and drink are prepared. Then gather the whole group together and place the covered tables in the centre of a large open space. Spread blankets around the area, away from the tables, and invite the children, four by four, to carry serving plates and cups of squash to the tables.

When everything is ready, give the children a plate each and explain that soon they can go to select food and a cup of drink to take to a blanket to sit and enjoy the feast. Then select two children and invite them to each choose a friend before going to fetch their food. Those two children then choose another two friends and so on, so that there is a continuous flow of children to the table.

Once the eating and drinking is over, gather everyone together and invite the children to take turns to tell the rest of the group about any new foods that they tried and whether they liked them or not.

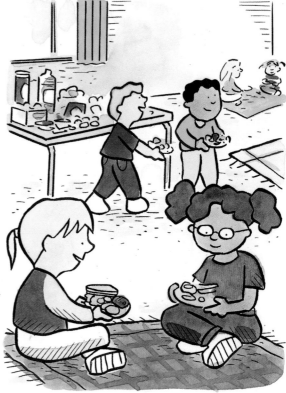

Support and extension
With very young children, ensure that you have an idea about their eating habits, so that you can provide at least one or two items that you know they will like. Invite older children to plan the menu with you and to make labels to go by each serving plate.

Home partnership
If any child tried something that they had never tasted before, celebrate this with their parents or carers at the end of the day.

Further ideas
♦ Hold a family picnic, where each family brings a small plate of food to put on the table for everyone to share.
♦ Set up the home corner as a café and encourage 'customers' to express their needs precisely.

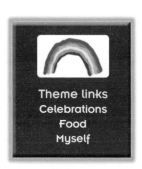
Theme links
Celebrations
Food
Myself

Foundation **Themes**
Senses

My party

Group size
Four children.

What you need
Tables; chairs; soft
toys; crockery;
cutlery.

What to do
Select a soft toy and tell the children
that it would like to have a tea party
with lots of friends. Invite each child
to choose a toy to invite and help the
group to set up the area accordingly.
Then join them at the table with
your toy.

As play progresses, invite the children to tell you about any parties that they
may have been to, asking them questions and comparing experiences. Discuss
the reasons for parties, where they are held and who might be invited. Notice
similarities, as well as differences, between the children's various experiences. Talk
about why your toy might have wanted a party and what the children think it might
like to do once it has eaten.

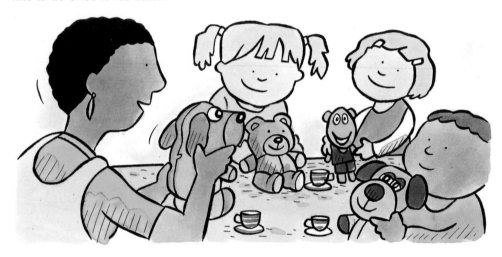

Ask what the children have done at parties, for example, played games, had
a bouncy castle or watched a conjurer. Encourage each child to recall their
experiences in sequence and in some detail, while the rest of the group supports
them by listening attentively.

Draw proceedings to a close by noticing that the toys are looking very tired and
ought to go home to bed. Encourage the guests and host to thank one another for a
lovely party and suggest that they might do it again some time.

Support and extension
Work with just one or two very young children at a time to maximise their
opportunities to speak. Encourage older children to ask questions of each other,
rather than doing this yourself.

Home partnership
Ask the children to bring in any photographs that they have of themselves at a party
to share with the group.

Further ideas
♦ Challenge the children to make a collage, using pictures cut from newspapers
and magazines, of people at parties.
♦ Invite the children to take turns to explain a party game that they know and, if
practical, play it together with the rest of the group.

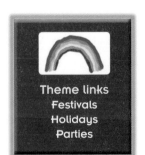

Theme links
Festivals
Holidays
Parties

Foundation
Themes
Senses

Sweet and sour

Group size
Six children.

What you need
Books about and pictures of the tongue; unbreakable mirrors; lemon juice; sugar; salt; other foodstuffs with distinctive flavours suitable for tasting; writing and drawing materials.

Check for any food allergies or dietary requirements.

What to do
Give each child a mirror and invite them to examine their tongue and compare it with the pictures in the books. Talk about the tongue and how it works. Give each child some sugar and invite them to taste a little and describe the sensation.

After a short discussion, put a label reading 'sweet' by the sugar and move on to the lemon juice. What can the children tell you about this taste? Invite them to look in the mirror as they taste the lemon juice on their tongues. Do they notice how their faces react?

After discussing the taste of the lemon, place a label reading 'sour' by the lemon juice, then move on to the salt and repeat the process, placing a 'salty' label in position. Then introduce the other foodstuffs and invite the children to select one for tasting. Encourage them to tell you what sort of flavour they think it has – sweet, sour or salty.

Most foods, of course, have complex flavours, and there will be no overriding taste, so opinions will vary, but explain to the children that there is no right or wrong. Invite them to experiment with the remaining foods, reminding them to use the mirrors sometimes to see if their faces can help them to decide upon a taste.

Support and extension
Support very young children by modelling words such as 'sweet', 'sour' and 'salty', and encourage them to use words other than 'nice' or 'bad' to describe the things that they taste. Encourage older children to record their experiments with drawings or writing.

Home partnership
Remind the children that they must never taste anything that they find without asking an adult first, because some things are dangerous to put in our mouths and might make us very ill. Ask parents and carers to reiterate this message at home.

Further ideas
♦ Investigate the agility of the tongue by waggling, stretching and curling it.
♦ Experiment by moving the tongue into different positions and noticing the effect that this has on your speech.
♦ Sing the song 'Sugar is sweet' on the photocopiable sheet on page 88 and read 'A riddle' on the photocopiable sheet on page 85 to the children.

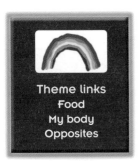

Theme links
Food
My body
Opposites

Foundation Themes
Senses

I like sausages!

Group size
Six to eight
children.

What you need
Paper plates; play
dough; pictures of
food; paints; acrylic
glue or varnish.

What to do

Tell the children that they are going to make a plate full of their favourite food using play dough. Talk about the colours of certain foods, for example: bananas are yellow, sausages are brown, peas are green, chips are yellow-brown and so on.

Demonstrate how to add a little paint to a ball of dough and how to knead it in to change the colour of the dough. Have the food pictures accessible for the children to refer to if necessary.

Before they begin, talk to each child about their favourite meal and help them decide how to start.

As the children work, discuss what they are trying to make and encourage them to think carefully about the shape, size and colour of the food that they are trying to model. When a child completes a piece of food, encourage them to compare it with the corresponding picture (if there is one) and make any necessary adjustments, before placing it on a paper plate to dry and beginning to make another item.

Once the children have completed their meals, leave these to dry and harden for several days.

Finally, coat each meal with varnish or clear acrylic glue to give a lasting finish.

Support and extension

It is useful to have some play food available for very young children to examine before they begin modelling their dough. Encourage older children to add details, such as gravy (brown paint) or a piece of lettuce (scrunched-up green tissue), to their plates for a touch of authenticity.

Home partnership

Exhibit the finished products with suitable captions and invite parents and carers to view them for a few days before letting the children take them home.

Further ideas

♦ Use the children's meals to set up a self-service café in the home corner.
♦ Act out the story of *Mrs Wobble the Waitress* by Allan Ahlberg (Puffin Books).

Theme links
Colours
Myself
Shapes

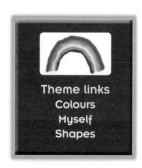

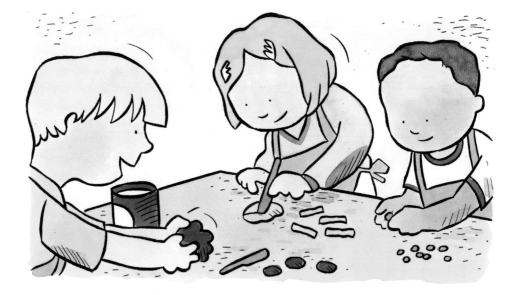

Pick a pizza

Group size
Up to eight children.

What you need
Yellow and red-pink sugar paper; bright red and green poster paper; scissors; glue; thick cardboard boxes; four shallow trays.

Preparation
Cut circles and squares (some big, some smaller) out of the cardboard boxes. Cut out the following paper shapes: yellow rectangles, bright red circles, green crescents and red-pink semicircles (with a larger diameter than the red circles). Put a few of the different shapes in separate trays, retaining the rest to replenish the trays later.

What to do
Look at the collage materials with the group and explain that they all go together to make a food beginning with 'p'. Place a cardboard base on the table and proceed to build up a pizza using the different coloured shapes, pausing intermittently to allow the children to guess what it is.

Once they have guessed correctly, congratulate them and stop making your pizza. Examine the coloured shapes together and talk about what they represent: yellow cheese rectangles, slices of red tomato, green pepper crescents and red-pink salami semicircles.

Look at the cardboard bases, talk about their different sizes and shapes, and explain that they can be used singly to make thin and crispy pizzas, or layered to make deep-pan pizzas. Invite the children to make pizzas of their own using the different 'ingredients'. Remind them to add their toppings evenly, so that everybody gets a bit of everything.

When a particular tray is empty, encourage the children to ask for replenishments using mathematical terms, for example, 'May we have more red circles, please?'. Leave completed pizzas to dry thoroughly before looking at them with the whole group and talking again about all the shapes and sizes.

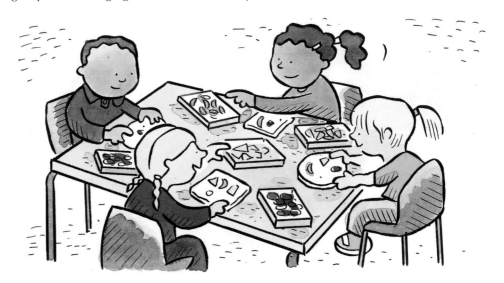

Support and extension
Remind very young children to glue the edges of their shapes and not just the middle. Encourage older children to cut out their own shapes and invent extras of their own, such as small, square flakes of tuna, or long, thin anchovy rectangles.

Home partnership
Ask parents and carers to help their children to notice and identify the different ingredients on any pizza that they have.

Further ideas
♦ Set up the interactive display 'Perfect pizzas' on page 81.
♦ Visit a pizza parlour, or invite in a pizza cook to demonstrate how the real thing is made.

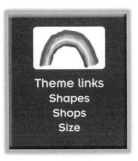

Theme links
Shapes
Shops
Size

Mealtime review

Stepping Stone
Complete a simple program on the computer and/or perform simple functions on ICT apparatus.

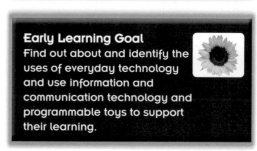

Early Learning Goal
Find out about and identify the uses of everyday technology and use information and communication technology and programmable toys to support their learning.

Group size
Whole group for the introduction and plenary, pairs of children for the activity.

What you need
A tape recorder; blank tape; microphone.

Preparation
Explain to the children that they are going to take it in turns to interview each other about the last meal that they ate. Talk about what an interview is and suitable questions to ask. Then invite two volunteers to begin, while the rest of the group follow other activities.

What to do
Talk to the two children about whom they might interview, helping them to formulate a few questions to ask. Demonstrate how to use the recorder and microphone. Allow a few minutes for them each to practise holding the microphone for the other to speak into, recording a few words and playing them back.

When they are familiar with the equipment, suggest that they set up an interviewing corner before inviting their first guest to the microphone. Let one child do the interviewing while the other acts as sound recordist, then change roles for the second guest. As they work, be ready to assist. Show them the 'pause' function for between questions to avoid long spaces.

Suggest to the children that they close each interview with a few words, for example, 'That was Natalie Huszar from Glen Hills Pre-school'. When one child has been interviewed, invite them to stay and watch the second interview before taking over as interviewer themselves.

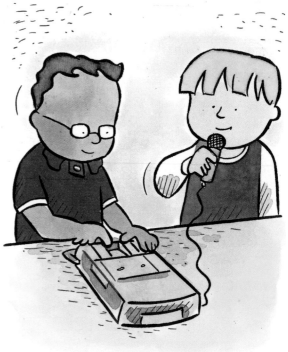

After two interviews, invite the sound recordists to rewind the tape for everyone to listen to. Let the interviewers choose alternative activities while you repeat the activity with the another pair. At the end of the session, gather the whole group together, listen to the entire tape and talk about what you have been doing.

Support and extension
Very young children may need considerable help to formulate relevant questions. Encourage older children to make notes or use pictures as an aide-mémoire, so that their interviews can flow smoothly.

Home partnership
Invite parents and carers to record one of their children's favourite stories or rhymes and bring it in to share with the group.

Further ideas
♦ Provide opportunities for the children to record one another using a still or video camera.
♦ Take the children to a local radio station or recording studio to see how things are done professionally.

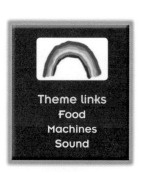

Theme links
Food
Machines
Sound

Carrots and cakes

Stepping Stone
Begin to use talk to pretend imaginary situations.

Early Learning Goal
Use language to imagine and re-create roles and experiences.

Group size
Six to eight children.

What you need
Sets of individual pictures, each showing a different foodstuff that starts with the same initial sound, such as cake, cauliflower, carrot; meat, marzipan, melon; chocolate, cheese, chips, and so on; samples of some of the foods shown; food-preparation equipment; tray; clean tea towel or similar; drawing and writing materials

Preparation
Prepare the food and place it on a covered tray for later.

Check for any food allergies or dietary requirements.

What to do
Look at each picture in turn and talk about what it is and the initial sound of its name. Then discuss which foods the children like and dislike, and talk about what they eat with them.

Next, challenge the children to find a pair of foods that begin with the same sound. Talk about the two foods chosen and ask the children what they think they might taste like if eaten together.

Put the pair of pictures to one side and repeat the challenge, again talking about the possible taste and encouraging each child to take a turn to speak. Once you have made as many pairs of pictures as you can, bring out your food samples.

Look at each pair of cards in turn, asking the children to tell you if they notice that you have a sample of *both* those foods on your tray. Invite the children to taste relevant pairs of foodstuffs for themselves to see whether their predictions about the combination were right.

Support and extension
Make the samples of food really tiny, by chopping or grating, to encourage very young children to try them. Invite older children to draw a selection of pairs of foods and write a few words about their combined taste.

Home partnership
Send home copies of the photocopiable sheet 'Food pairs' on page 94 and encourage parents and carers to continue the activity with their children.

Further ideas
♦ Develop the children's imaginative thinking by reading the first part of a story and challenging them to finish it.
♦ Encourage creative thinking by frequently asking the children, 'What if...?' questions, for example, 'What if milk came out of our taps instead of water?' or 'What if we walked on our hands instead of our feet?'.

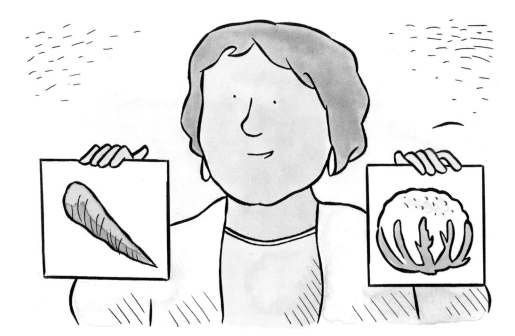

Theme links
Healthy eating
Pairs
Things I like

Foundation Themes
Senses

Rainbow mints

Group size
Up to six children.

What you need
Fondant icing; peppermint essence; food colourings; aprons; flat trays or plates.

Preparation
Ensure that all surfaces are hygienically clean.

Check for any food allergies or dietary requirements.

What to do
Explain to the children that they are going to make some peppermint creams to share with the rest of the group. Ensure that they wash their hands thoroughly, then put on aprons, push up sleeves and give the children a small piece of fondant icing each (about the size of a kiwi fruit).

Invite each child to knead the icing to soften it, before rolling it into a ball and making a deep indentation in the top with their finger. Put a couple of drops of peppermint essence into the indentation and again invite the children to knead the icing thoroughly before rolling it back into a ball. Introduce the food colourings and explain to the children that they are allowed to choose either one or two colours to put into their icing.

Once they have chosen, suggest that they make either one or two indentations for the colourings. Give each child two drops of colouring of their choice and again ask them to knead the dough thoroughly. As they work, encourage them to talk about what they see happening. Look at the colours as they mix and notice the depths and tones as they develop.

When the children are satisfied with their icing, show them how to break off small pieces, roll them into balls and flatten them to make round sweets. Leave these in a cool place to harden for an hour or two, before sharing them with the rest of the group. Wash hands thoroughly, noticing what happens to the soap!

Support and extension
Work with only one or two very young children at a time to ensure conditions are kept as hygienic as possible. Challenge older children to make different-shaped sweets, including flowers, hearts and stars.

Home partnership
Put aside a few creams for each child to take home to share with their families.

Further ideas
♦ Provide different-coloured fruit squash and notice what happens when it is poured into different-coloured cups.
♦ Make pictures using cooked spaghetti dyed different colours.

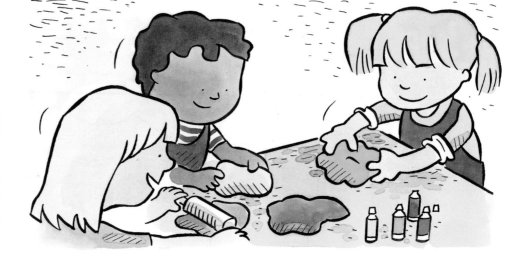

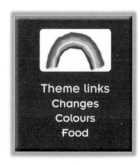

Theme links
Changes
Colours
Food

Chapter 5

Smell

This chapter contains activities to help children select their own tools and equipment and handle them safely, to count reliably, and to extend their vocabulary as they enjoy opportunities to make greetings cards and books, act out a favourite story and explore a sensory sand tray.

Sensory sand

Group size
Six children.

What you need
Table; small, deep trays; dry sand; selection of herbs or essences, such as lavender, sage, rose and peppermint; small funnels, sieves, spoons and pots; dustpans and brushes; water; lidded containers; eye-droppers; scissors.

Preparation
Pour sand into each of the trays and add a different scent to each one. Fill the lidded containers with scented water or chopped leaves to match the trays.

What to do
Encourage the children to talk about the smell from each tray and discuss any thoughts or memories that it might trigger. Then invite each child to select a tray and a few tools, and observe them as they tip and pour the sand.

After a while, pause the activity and ask the children if they want to continue using the same tray or whether they would like to swap with a friend to experience a different scent. Suggest that, before they continue the activity, they sweep up any loose sand. Demonstrate how to use the dustpan efficiently, letting each child sweep up their own sand before carrying on.

After several minutes, pause the activity again and ask the children if they can still smell their sand or if it is losing its potency. If the scent needs refreshing, encourage the group to compare smells to decide which container of scented water should be used for each tray.

Invite each child to use an eye-dropper to transfer a few drops of the appropriate water, or scissors to chop leaves, into their tray. Continue the activity for a few more minutes, before finishing by sweeping up spills and asking each child to ask a friend to make a new group to repeat the activity.

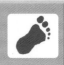

Stepping Stone
Use one-handed tools and equipment.

Early Learning Goal
Handle tools, objects, construction and malleable materials safely and with increasing control.

Support and extension
Hold the dustpan for very young children while they sweep up their sand. Encourage older children to sieve their spilt sand to remove debris, before pouring it back into their tray.

Home partnership
Encourage parents and carers to help develop their children's co-ordination skills by letting them practise sweeping up leaves and other garden debris.

Further ideas
♦ Arrange regular cleaning sessions, so that the children can practise their skills with dusters, mops, shoe-brushes, brooms, scrubbing brushes and other simple tools.
♦ Provide a shallow tray full of gravel and a selection of hoes, rakes and sticks for pattern-making activities.

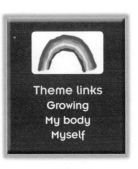

Theme links
Growing
My body
Myself

Fantastic flowers

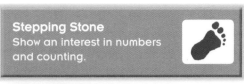
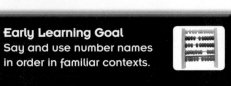
Group size
Four to eight children.

What you need
Strips of tissue paper (at least 10cm x 60cm) in two different colours; thin garden sticks in three different lengths; sticky tape; scissors; perfumes; cotton wool; glue; pots of sand.

What to do

Tell the group that you are going to make some beautiful fragrant flowers, and invite each child to select some coloured tissue to work with. Demonstrate how to gather, fold or scrunch the paper together along one edge, leaving the other edge to fan out to make a flower. Explain how to push a stick down through the centre of the flower and secure it with tape to make a stalk, before adding a ball of perfumed cotton wool to its centre.

As the children work, encourage them to each think about the size and shape of their flower and have scissors available, so that they can shape the edge to make frills or petals if desired. Invite them to look at the different sticks and decide which length might suit their flower-head best.

When each child has completed their basic flower, give them a small ball of perfumed cotton wool to glue in the centre. Spend some time counting the finished flowers (forwards, backwards, in pairs and by colour) and sort them into the pots by colour or height.

Invite the children to make another flower each to add to the stock, perhaps using different colours this time. Use all the completed flowers for counting, sorting and ordering activities based on colour, height and smell.

Support and extension

With very young children, work with a group size of up to four. Encourage older children to set problems for each other, such as, 'How many more red flowers than blue flowers are there?'.

Home partnership

Encourage parents and carers to help their children to see how many flowers they can count on the way home.

Further ideas

♦ Use the photocopiable sheet 'Sunflowers' on page 95 for more counting practice.
♦ Go for a walk to see how many blue, red or orange flowers you can spot.

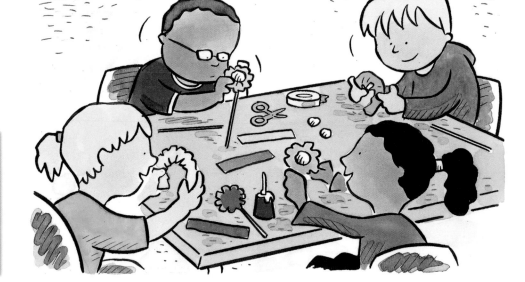

Theme links
Colours
Growing
Size

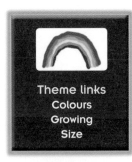

Foundation Themes
Senses

Spicy pictures

Stepping Stone
Understand that equipment and tools have to be used safely.

Early Learning Goal
Handle tools, objects, construction and malleable materials safely and with increasing control.

Group size
Four to six children.

What you need
A selection of herbs and spices of different shapes and colours, such as bay leaves, cloves, cinnamon sticks, caraway and cardamom seeds; glue and brushes; pairs of tweezers; 15cm paper circles; small spoons.

What to do

Look at the herbs and spices together and discuss the different aromas, shapes and colours. Explain to the children that they are going to make pictures using those things. Look at the tweezers and talk about how they work and what they might be used for.

Explain that the tweezers must be used carefully and sensibly to avoid nipping flesh in them. Demonstrate how to brush glue thickly on to a paper circle and place a cardamom seed on it using tweezers.

Invite the children to practise picking up and carrying various objects with tweezers, before beginning their pictures. As they work, notice who is having difficulty using the tweezers and be ready to offer verbal encouragement and assistance if necessary.

Continue to talk about the smells of the ingredients and how they blend together to make new smells. Display the finished pictures alongside the ingredients, so that others can identify and match what was used where.

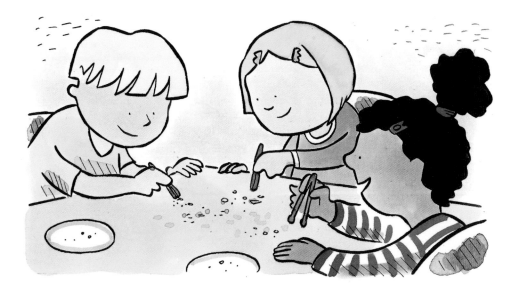

Support and extension

If very young children find tweezers too difficult to manipulate, provide small spoons instead. Encourage older children to explain what they intend to do before they begin and to talk about how satisfied they are with the result.

Home partnership

Ask parents and carers to donate interesting items to add to your natural collage collection, for example, pistachio shells, clean eggshells, linseed, green and orange lentils, black rice and so on.

Further ideas

♦ Regularly change the tools and equipment in your craft area to include less common items, such as a manual paper shredder, single hole-punch, paper crinkler or embossed rollers.

♦ Set up a supervised woodworking area to safely introduce the children to hammers and nails, or screws and screwdrivers.

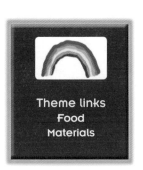

Theme links
Food
Materials

Foundation Themes
Senses

Flowers for sale

Stepping Stone
Use some number names accurately in play.

Early Learning Goal
Count reliably up to 10 everyday objects.

Group size
Up to four children.

What you need
Artificial flowers sprayed with perfume (or use the flowers made in the activity 'Fantastic flowers' on page 64); pots of sand; table; cash register; pennies; purses; wrapping paper; writing materials; price labels; 2p, 5p and 10p coins.

What to do
Gather the group together to smell the flowers, look at the pots of sand, the cash register, labels, purses and paper and discuss what they might be for. Lead the children to discover that you are going to set up a flower shop or stall and talk about how this might be done.

Involve the children in counting out the flowers in sets to put in the pots and arranging the rest of the equipment. Look at the numbers on the price labels and practise counting out the correct number of pennies for each one, before placing the labels by the pots.

Let the children take turns to be the stallholder. Play alongside the shoppers, encouraging them to choose which flowers they want by smelling them and considering both their colour and size. Remind them that they must tell the stallholder how many they want of each and that they have to count out enough pennies for each one. The stallholder must then wrap the flowers and check the proffered money carefully.

At the end of the session, help the children to tidy the shop by sorting and counting the flowers into the pots and counting the pennies into the cash register and purses.

Support and extension
Price every flower at one penny for very young children. Provide a variety of coins for older children, so that they can practise giving and receiving change.

Home partnership
Appeal to parents and carers for any unwanted artificial plants and flowers that they might be willing to donate to your stall.

Further ideas
♦ Instead of 'Five Currant Buns' (Traditional), sing and act out: 'Five pretty flowers in the shop to sell. Beautiful colours and what a lovely smell. Along came (child's name) with a penny one day, bought a pretty flower and took it away'.
♦ Invite the children to examine empty grocery packaging to discover how many cakes, eggs or chocolates it originally contained.

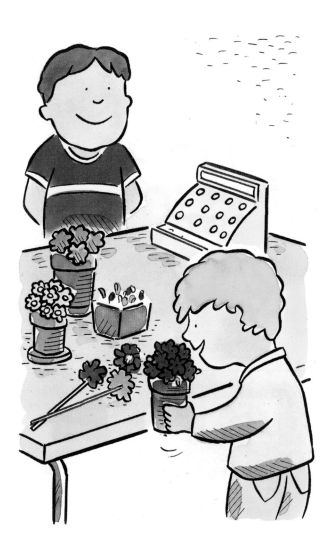

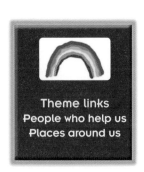
Theme links
People who help us
Places around us

Our book of noses

Group size
Up to eight children.

What you need
Scissors; old magazines containing a variety of animal and human faces; stiff paper; writing materials; glue; stapler or sticky tape; mirror card.

Preparation
Separate the pages of the magazines, discarding those showing no faces. Staple or glue the stiff paper together to make a blank zigzag or conventional book.

What to do
Explain that you are going to make a book about noses and ask the children what they know about them. Ask them what noses are for and what they can do. Show them the blank book and explain that you will need a lot of pictures to go inside. Give each child a page from the magazines and ask them to find a nose.

Help the children to describe the noses that they have found, using a wide vocabulary and introducing words such as 'wrinkly', 'twitchy' or 'narrow'. If some of the noses are a bit too similar, suggest that the children select a better variety from the pages that you have available. Invite each child to cut out their chosen face complete with nose, put it aside for later use and select another one to cut out.

While the group continues to work, invite one child at a time to paste a nose or two into the book, leaving space for captions and the last page empty. When the book is finished, gather the group together and decide on a suitable caption for each page, for example, 'long nose' (elephant), 'short nose' (mouse), 'twitchy nose' (rabbit), 'runny nose' (child), 'red nose' (clown) and so on.

Ensure that the whole group can observe as you write each caption and say the words. Paste a sheet of mirror card on the last page and silently write 'my nose' under it. Help the children to read what it says. Finally, read the whole book through together, passing it from child to child to read the last page.

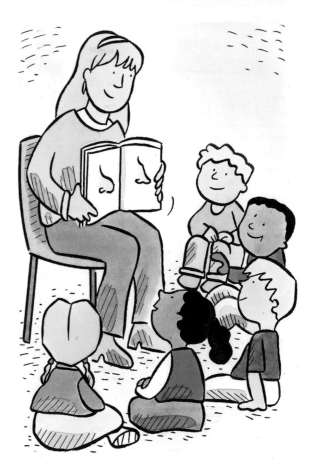

Support and extension
Draw a guiding line to help very young children to each cut around the outline of their chosen face. Encourage older children to write their own captions.

Home partnership
Invite the children to tell their parents and carers what they have been doing and to ask them to look at the book of noses before they go home.

Further ideas
♦ Set up the interactive display 'Noses' on page 82.
♦ Learn the rhyme 'My nose' on the photocopiable sheet on page 85.

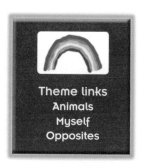

Theme links
Animals
Myself
Opposites

Foundation
Themes
Senses

It's a lemon!

Stepping Stone
Examine objects and living things to find out more about them.

Early Learning Goal
Investigate objects and materials by using all of their senses as appropriate.

Group size
Six children.

What you need
Lidded film canisters; awl (adult use); two each of a selection of foodstuffs with distinctive aromas, such as a lemon, onion, garlic, cloves, peppermints, sardines and sage.

Preparation
Keep one of each item intact for later use. Then, enclose a small amount of each matching item in a separate canister and pierce holes in the lid to allow the aroma to escape.

What to do
Look at the intact foodstuffs together in turn, handling them, smelling them and talking about their texture, shape and aroma. Arrange them in a line and run through them again, naming them and giving a few descriptive words about each one.

Then introduce the canisters, explaining to the children that they are going to play a game to try to find out what is inside the pots without looking. How do the children think they will be able to do that? Pass a canister around for them to handle and lead them to discover that they can smell the contents.

Invite a volunteer to be first to play the game. Give them a canister and challenge them to sniff it and then find the item with the matching smell. When they have selected one, take the lid off the pot, look at its contents and decide whether it is correct. If it is, the volunteer can choose the next person to play; if not, you choose. Replace the lid on the canister, return the item to the display and continue the game until everyone has had at least one turn.

At the end of the activity, ensure that everyone washes their hands thoroughly to avoid irritations from the foodstuffs.

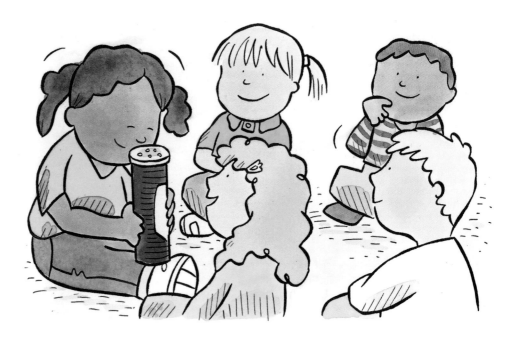

Support and extension
For younger children, work with no more than two children at a time. Encourage older children to organise the game themselves, with minimal support, but do remind them to wash their hands at the end.

Home partnership
Explain to parents and carers what you have been doing and encourage them to play 'Guess the smell' games at home.

Further ideas
♦ Sing the song 'I can smell' on the photocopiable sheet on page 88.
♦ Go to the local library to find books and stories about smells and smelling.

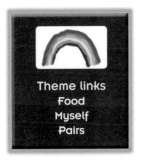

Theme links
Food
Myself
Pairs

A present for someone special

Stepping Stone
Persist for extended periods of time at an activity of their choosing.

Early Learning Goal
Maintain attention, concentrate, and sit quietly when appropriate.

Group size
Four children.

What you need
A small orange or lemon for each child; lengths of ribbon; cloves; sections of cardboard tube; sharp knife (adult use); writing materials; sturdy twig set in a pot of sand or gravel.

Preparation
Make a sample pomander, following the instructions in 'What to do'.

What to do
Show the pomander to the group and explain that, many years ago, people used to carry around pomanders made from special herbs and spices to ward off germs. Explain that they could also be used to perfume rooms or wardrobes, because people did not have all the sprays and household perfumes that we have today.

Pass the pomander around for the children to handle and smell, encouraging them to share their thoughts about it. Ask them to think about someone that they know who might like a pomander as a present, such as Mum, Grandma, a brother or a friend.

Invite the children to select either an orange or a lemon, a cardboard-tube stand for the fruit and two lengths of ribbon. If a lemon is particularly pointed, cut off the ends to make it simpler for the ribbon to lie flat. Help each child to tie their ribbons securely around their fruit, dividing it into four sections, and to leave a hanging loop at the top.

Encourage each child to rest their fruit on its stand while they stud it all over with cloves, placing them as close or as spaced as they wish. Label the finished items and suspend them from the twig for a few days before sending them home.

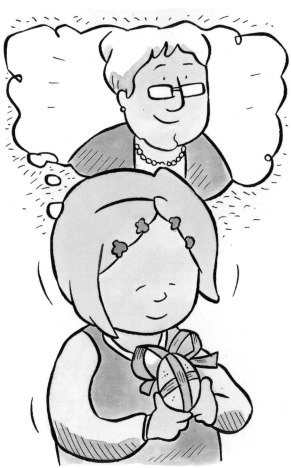

Support and extension
If very young children find it difficult to maintain attention to complete the task, suggest that they leave it for a while and come back later to continue. Encourage older children to each make and attach a gift label to their pomander.

Home partnership
Send home the pomanders to be given as gifts.

Further ideas
♦ Invite in local artisans to demonstrate their craft, such as origami, pottery, kite-making and so on.
♦ Arrange a series of story sessions at your local library, gradually increasing their length as the children's concentration develops.

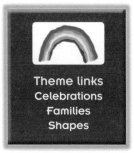

Theme links
Celebrations
Families
Shapes

Scented gardens

Group size
Six to eight children.

What you need
Shallow trays of damp sand; tiny twigs; gravel; mirror card; cotton wool; cotton buds; tissue paper; perfumes; glue; scissors.

Preparation
Ensure that that all the children have had previous experience of working freely with art and craft materials. Prepare a few sample trees and flowers by decorating twigs and cotton buds with tissue paper. Put the perfumes to one side until later.

What to do
Spend some time talking about gardens and the things found in them, such as trees, flowers, paths, ponds and so on, and the different scents produced by some plants. Tell the children that they are going to make gardens of their own, using the materials available.

Show the children your sample trees and flowers and explain that they are examples to give them ideas of their own. Demonstrate how to 'plant' them in the damp sand. Give the children the trays of sand and invite them to select their materials and start work.

Encourage the children to think and talk about what they are doing. Ask them questions, such as 'Will there be a path in the garden?', 'What time of year is it?', 'What colour might the leaves be?', 'Is it a fantasy garden, where anything is possible?' and so on.

When the gardens are nearing completion, invite the children to look carefully to see if there is anything that they want to rearrange, add or remove.

Once they are all happy with their creations, ask them to think again about gardens and help them to remember what you talked about at the beginning. Remind them that some plants do not just *look* attractive, they also have different scents. Then introduce the perfumes and invite the children to sprinkle small amounts on some of their plants to complete their gardens.

Support and extension
Use dropper perfume bottles with very young children to avoid over-liberal application. With older childre, use larger trays and encourage them to work in pairs, rather than individually.

Home partnership
Give each child a copy of the photocopiable sheet 'My garden' on page 96 and encourage them to complete it at home, using whatever materials that they have available, and to bring it back to show the group.

Further ideas
♦ Use natural materials outside to make temporary sculptures or pictures.
♦ Build an ongoing group sculpture from recyclable materials, adding pieces and changing its structure at will.

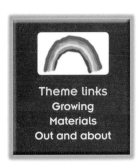

Theme links
Growing
Materials
Out and about

Foundation Themes
Senses

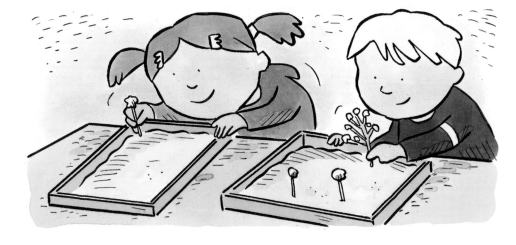

I smell breakfast!

What to do
Talk with the children about smells that they like and dislike. Encourage them to try to say why they feel the way they do about a particular smell. Ask if it reminds them of something that they did or somewhere they went in the past.

Explain that often smells do remind people of certain things, and share some of your own memory smells with the children. Invite the group to take turns to talk about a smell that evokes particular memories for them.

Then tell the children that you have brought a few smells with you to see if they remind anyone of anything. Ask for a volunteer to wear the blindfold and take the first sniff. Use the fabric to conceal the item or canister from the group while you waft it under the volunteer's nose. Let them talk about any memory that it brings to them, before inviting a second volunteer to take a turn. Continue the activity, using different items and volunteers, until everyone who wants to has had a turn.

Finally, reveal each item in turn and leave all the smells accessible for the children to use again in their own time.

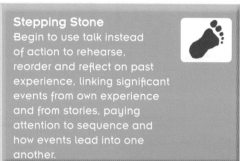

Stepping Stone
Begin to use talk instead of action to rehearse, reorder and reflect on past experience, linking significant events from own experience and from stories, paying attention to sequence and how events lead into one another.

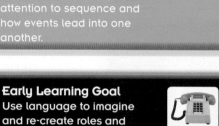

Early Learning Goal
Use language to imagine and re-create roles and experiences.

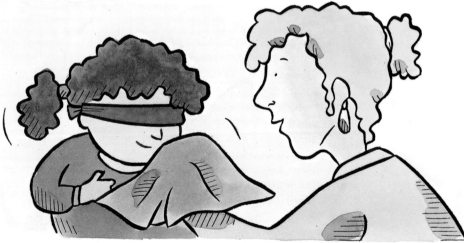

Support and extension
Very young children may prefer not to be blindfolded, so use the card as a screen instead. Encourage older children to write or dictate a few words about any object that evokes memories for them.

Home partnership
Explain to parents and carers what you have been doing and encourage them to share some of their own anecdotes about memory-evoking smells with their children.

Further ideas
♦ Ask the children to show the rest of the group an object from home that brings back memories to them.
♦ Go for a walk in the local area, stopping at various points to read signs or look at interesting features, such as fire hydrants. When you return, try to recall where you went and what you did.

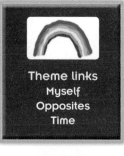

Theme links
Myself
Opposites
Time

Foundation Themes
Senses

A card for Mum

Group size
Four to six children.

What you need
Coloured card, scored and folded in half; tissue paper; coloured cotton wool; scissors; glue; sticky tape; writing equipment; floral perfume oils such as geranium, jasmine, lavender, rose and so on.

What to do
Tell the children that they are going to make pretty flower cards for their mums and that they will be very special flowers because they will be perfumed too – just like some real flowers. Remain sensitive to individual children's circumstances and suggest to them that they make their card for another significant female, if appropriate.

Early Learning Goal
Select the tools and techniques they need to shape, assemble and join materials they are using.

Put one drop of each oil on small pieces of cotton wool and pass them around the group for them to smell. Explain that the perfume will be the last thing that goes on their card and suggest that the first thing to do might be to write the greetings inside. Talk about why this is the case and lead the children to realise that once the card has glue and a flower on it, it will be difficult to open and write on.

Once all the greetings are complete, invite each child to think about their flower: will it have a stalk and what colour will it be? Ask them to think about its shape and its number of petals. Encourage them to think about how they will cut, fold and arrange the materials to make a flower, reminding them that the perfumed cotton wool will need to go in the centre of their flower to complete it.

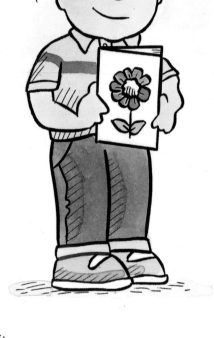

Observe the children as they work and be ready to give advice and practical assistance if required. When their card is complete, let each child choose a perfumed cotton-wool ball and paste it into position in the centre of their flower.

Support and extension
Supply very young children with a variety of ready-cut petals rather than expecting them to cut their own. Encourage older children to each make an envelope to encase their card.

Home partnership
Send home the cards to be given to mums or special people.

Further ideas
♦ Challenge the children to each make a bed for a favourite toy, using their own choice of items from the recyclable-materials box.
♦ Invite the children to each make themselves a hat, from whatever materials they want, and hold a fashion parade to show off the results.

Theme links
Celebrations
My family
Shapes

Follow your nose

Early Learning Goal
Understand what is right, what is wrong, and why.

Group size
Six children.

What you need
An outdoor area with a variety of smells, such as plants and herbs, new-mown grass, bonfire smoke and so on; card; marker pens.

Preparation
Plan a route to follow that will lead you past as many different aromas as possible. Using the card and marker pen, draw a picture of a large nose for each different aroma, plus an extra one. Place a picture of a nose by each aromatic point and add an arrow pointing towards the next one along the route.

What to do
Ensure that all the children are properly clad (and have been to the toilet!). Explain that, when they are outside, they must all stay together and listen carefully to what is being said.

Once outdoors, tell the children that they are going to play a game called 'Follow your nose', then show them the spare picture of a nose. Ask them if they can spot another nose picture anywhere, and when they do, walk towards it, talking about what it might be for.

When they arrive at the designated spot, invite the children to guess why it might be there and lead them to discover that it tells them that there is something here to smell. Once the group has smelled and discussed the item or area, draw the children's attention to the arrow and decide what it indicates.

Continue to follow the noses along the planned route, but, if an unexpected smell wafts by, stop to savour that, too. When you are back at the setting, try to recall all the different objects that you smelled on your walk.

Support and extension
Partner a very young child with an adult or a more mature child, until they are aware of the behavioural boundaries set. Encourage older children to repeat the trail, acting as guide to a friend who has not already experienced it.

Home partnership
Encourage parents and carers to help their children to notice and identify different smells both on the journey home and in their houses.

Further ideas
♦ Take groups of children to a local shop to buy ingredients for a cooking session.
♦ Invite the local road safety officer in to talk to the group.

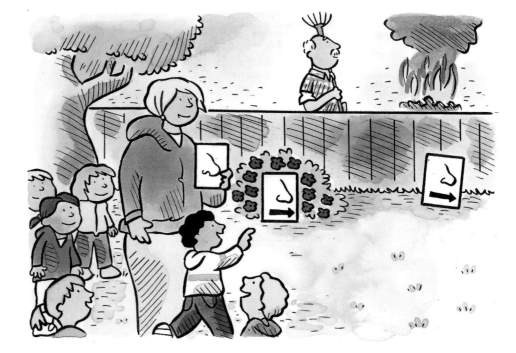

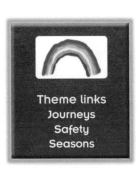

Theme links
Journeys
Safety
Seasons

Foundation Themes
Senses

I smell boy!

Group size
Whole group.

What you need
A copy of 'Jack and the Beanstalk' (Traditional); space to move around in safety.

Preparation
Read or tell the story of 'Jack and the Beanstalk' to ensure that the children are familiar with it.

What to do
Tell the children that they are going to act out the story of Jack and recall the main events in order.

Spread out around the room and warm up by practising some key movements, such as climbing the beanstalk, curling up small to hide, striding like a giant, creeping away softly, running and chopping down the beanstalk.

Begin to tell the story, taking the part of Jack's mother and encouraging the children to reply in character as Jack. Encourage them to move around the room appropriately, by incorporating a variety of action words into the narrative, for example, 'Jack *skipped* along towards the market'.

Continue to play the minor characters yourself, while the children play the part of Jack, joining in verbally wherever appropriate. Once in the castle, invite the children to alternately take the part of Jack and of the giant, emphasising the parts about smelling 'the blood of an Englishman'.

When it comes to the final chase, switch the narrative back and forth between the main characters, for example, 'Jack ran and ran on his little legs and the giant came pounding along with great big strides', while the children change character appropriately. At the end of the story, invite the whole group to say the final line: 'And Jack and his mother were never poor again'.

Support and extension
Be aware that some very young children could become frightened if they are surrounded by particularly 'fierce giants', so be ready to partner them with a friend or adult for support. With older children, divide the group up, so that each section plays a different role.

Home partnership
Ask the children to bring in a favourite story from home to share with the group.

Further ideas
♦ Provide a drama corner stocked with favourite tales, where the children can act out the stories in their own time.
♦ Visit a local theatre with the children to see a show, or invite in a theatre group to perform for the children.

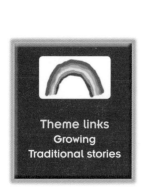

Theme links
Growing
Traditional stories

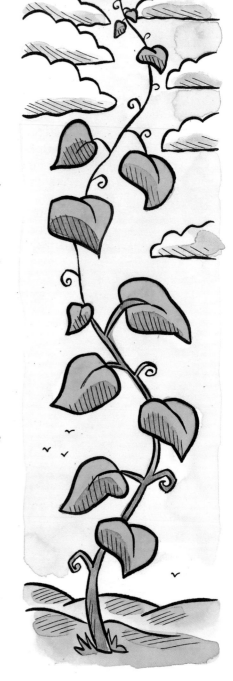

Circle time

Circle-time activities are designed for the whole group, providing opportunities for the children to interact and to work as part of a team. The activities increase the children's ability to communicate effectively and to learn to share tasks.

I can see

What to do
Sit with the children in an inward-facing circle, holding the ball in your lap. Explain to the group that you are going to describe someone and that they are going to have to try to guess who it is. If a child guesses correctly, you will roll the ball gently across the circle to them, but if they cannot guess, you will have to choose a different child and start again.

Remind the children to listen carefully to what you say and to look at each of the other children in the circle to find the one matching your description. Look around the circle, select a child and begin to describe them (without looking directly at them), for example, 'I can see a girl and she has long, blond hair'.

Once someone has guessed which child you have described, roll the ball gently to them and invite them to continue the activity, by choosing a different child, describing them and rolling the ball to the person who has guessed correctly. Encourage the speaker to talk loudly enough for everyone to hear and to use whole sentences for their description, gradually adding more information to enable a correct identification to be made.

As play continues, ask the child with the ball to try to choose a child who has not had a turn yet. Once everybody has had a turn, spend a few moments freely rolling the ball back and forth among the group, calling the name of the intended recipient as you send the ball on its way.

Stepping Stone
Use language for an increasing range of purposes.

Early Learning Goal
Speak clearly and audibly with confidence and control and show awareness of the listener, for example by their use of conventions such as greetings, 'please' and 'thank you'.

Further ideas
♦ Vary the game by having one child issuing instructions and another rolling the ball, for example, 'Roll the ball to a boy wearing a blue jumper'. If they follow the instructions correctly, the instructor rolls the next ball while the child who received the ball becomes the instructor. If they are wrong, the recipient of the ball becomes the roller and the instructor tries again.
♦ Play a game of 'Guess what?' with the children by taking turns to hide an object under a cloth in the centre of the circle and describing it until someone identifies it correctly.

Don't drop it!

What to do

Stand the children in a circle facing outwards and give the beanbag to one of them. Explain that they are going to pass the beanbag around the circle without dropping it. If it does fall to the floor, then it must be taken back to its starting-point. Invite the child with the beanbag to start the game.

When a circuit has been completed successfully, congratulate the children and challenge them to repeat the activity, this time using only one hand. Praise their success and challenge them to do it now with their eyes closed – first with two hands and then with only one – so that they must feel for the beanbag rather than watch for it.

Again, congratulate them on their success and challenge them to repeat it again, now passing the beanbag behind their backs without looking. Remind them to use their hands to feel where the next child's hands are and not to let go of the beanbag until the other child is holding it firmly. Continue to challenge them further, by asking them to use their feet to pass the beanbag or to pass it alternately in front of, and then behind, them around the circle.

Next, invite the children to take turns to invent new rules for passing the beanbag, then try some of the ideas out and discuss their level of difficulty. Finish the session by asking the children to think about what they have been doing and to try to invent some similar games to play among themselves.

Further ideas

◆ Sew familiar objects, such as a comb, spoon, wooden cube and coin, inside small black cloth bags, put them inside a box and pass the box to different children in turn, asking them to feel the bags and find a named object, continuing until the box is empty.

◆ Make a circle of string with a curtain ring threaded on it for the group to surreptitiously pass around under their hands, while a volunteer in the centre of the circle tries to guess where it is.

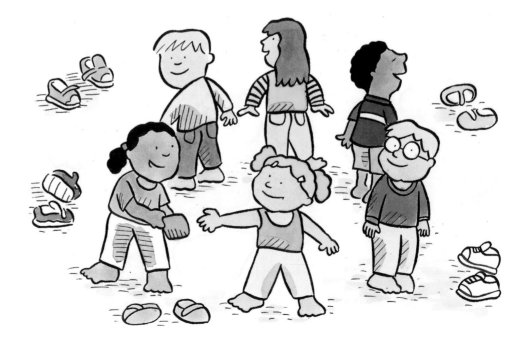

Pass the bells

Stepping Stone
Begin to move rhythmically.

Early Learning Goal
Recognise and explore how sounds can be changed, sing simple songs from memory, recognise repeated sounds and sound patterns and match movement to music.

What you need
Bells.

What to do

Sit the group in an inward-facing circle and introduce the bells. Ask the children to pass them all the way around the circle without making a sound. Then demonstrate how different rhythms can be achieved by shaking the bells a number of times, resting and shaking them again to make a pattern of sound. Choose a simple rhythmic pattern, for example, two shakes, rest, two shakes, rest. Talk about it with the children, encouraging them to keep the rhythm themselves by repeatedly clapping twice and stopping in time to the bells. Let each child have a turn to reproduce the rhythm, using bells as well as clapping.

Once the children are familiar with the idea, challenge them to make the pattern as they pass the bells around the circle again, so each child shakes the bells twice and silently passes them to the next to create a rest before the next child repeats the action.

Support the group initially, by quietly clapping the rhythm or verbalising it – 'Shake, shake, pass, shake, shake, pass' – but gradually withdraw the support until the children are able to keep the rhythm going themselves. Encourage the children to keep the same rhythm while the bells are passed all the way around the circle, then in reverse back to the start.

Next, introduce different rhythms, making them as complex or as simple as necessary to suit the group. Be ready to support verbally or with clapping at any time to maintain the rhythm. Try the activity with different instruments, for example, a drum, chime bar and shaker.

Finally, close the activity by passing the bells around the circle trying to keep them ringing the whole time, with no break in the sound at all.

Further ideas

♦ Record some continuous simple rhythms lasting several minutes and use them to stimulate pattern-painting or movement sequences.
♦ Make a collection of rhythms from different countries or cultures and have them accessible for the children to listen and move freely to, either indoors or outdoors.

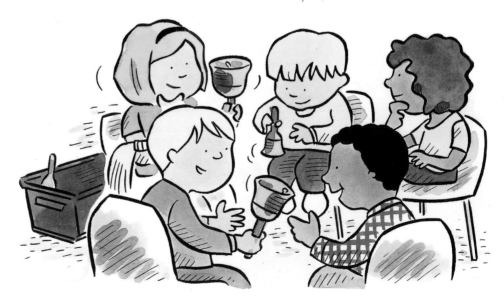

Fruit salad

What you need
A selection of
different fruit
in a bag; tray;
hygienic food
preparation
and serving
equipment; cloth;
two adults.

Check for any food
allergies or dietary
requirements.

What to do
Put the tray in the centre of the circle
and hold the bag of fruit, while the
second adult remains near by, ready
to prepare the fruit as the game
progresses. Select one fruit and show it to the group. Talk about what it is, which
country it might be grown in and what it is called. Place it on the tray and choose a
second fruit.

Continue in this way until seven or eight different pieces of fruit are on the tray.
Explain that you are going to cover the fruit in a minute, and secretly take one away to
see if the children can guess which one you have taken. Point to each fruit in turn and
check that the children know its name, before covering all the fruit with the cloth.

Remove one fruit as you uncover the tray and invite the children to put up
their hands if they think that they can tell you what you have taken. If they cannot
remember the name of the fruit, ask them to describe it instead and ask the rest of
the group to help with the name. If they are right, give the fruit to the other adult to
prepare and place in a bowl to begin a fruit salad. If they are wrong, return the fruit
to the tray and try again.

Once all the pieces of fruit have been guessed and prepared, share the resulting
salad among the group, encouraging them to identify the various pieces as they eat
them and to try to remember what each looked like before it was prepared.

Further ideas
♦ Play blindfold tasting games with fruit or cooked vegetables, giving the player a
whole, unprepared fruit or vegetable as a clue if they cannot make an identification
through taste alone.
♦ Share *Ketchup on Your Cornflakes?* by Nick Sharratt (Scholastic) and talk about
the possible tastes of the various combinations of food that it contains.

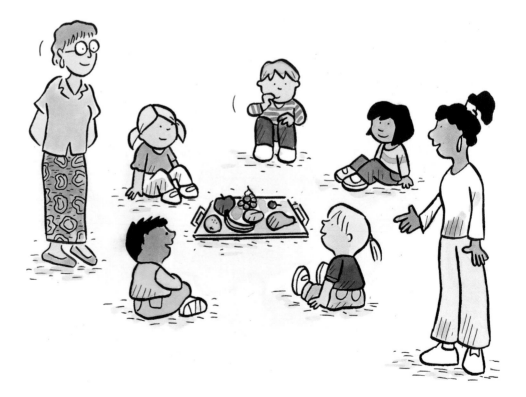

Displays

This section gives suggestions for four interactive displays, each focusing on one of the senses and related to particular activities described in the relevant chapters.

Patterns

What to do
Look at the kaleidoscopes together. Talk about the way that smaller patterns are repeated to make a large circular pattern, then introduce the paper snowflake, noticing the similar patterns as those seen inside a kaleidoscope. Fold and unfold the paper so that the children can see how the pattern was made. Display the pattern on the wall and ask for their advice as to where to place it.

Now invite the group to use the materials on the craft table to make patterns for the wall. Gradually build up the display, adding a title or caption, such as 'Patterns'.

Once the wall is complete, demonstrate to the group how to use Blu-Tack to stick three mirrors together along their edges to make a kaleidoscope with which to view the world around them and invite them to try it for themselves.

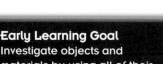
Stepping Stone
Examine objects and living things to find out more about them.

Early Learning Goal
Investigate objects and materials by using all of their senses as appropriate.

Using the display
♦ Ask the children to experiment with the paper circles to make a variety of patterns.
♦ Encourage the children to experiment with the mirrors to make square or pentagonal kaleidoscopes and talk about the effects.

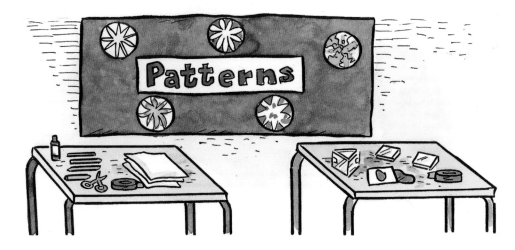

Changing sounds

Early Learning Goal
Recognise and explore how
sounds can be changed, sing
simple songs from memory,
recognise repeated sounds
and sound patterns and match
movements to music.

What you need
Art, craft and writing
materials; frieze
paper; selection
of real and child-
made instruments
(see the activity
'Crash, twang,
boom!' on page
40); two tables;
tape recorder;
songbooks.

Preparation
Back the wall with
frieze paper and
add a border of
black musical notes
on white paper.
Put one table in
front of the display,
placing containing
real instruments
on it, such as
cymbals, drums,
chime bars, small
guitars, shakers
and scrapers.
Leave the second
table, displaying
the child-made
instruments, to one
side.

What to do
Invite the children to take turns to choose an instrument from those on the display table and draw or paint a large picture of it to cut out and go on the wall. Once the pictures are in position, help the children to produce 'sound word' labels to display among them, such as 'boom', 'twang', 'squeal', 'crash' and so on.

Add the second table to the first to give a large display area for both the real and the home-made instruments.

Using the display
♦ Encourage the children to experiment with different instruments to see how many sounds they can produce. Play a simple rhythm on one instrument and challenge the children to copy or continue it on an instrument of their choosing.
♦ Ask the children to invent their own rhythms or make up songs to sing together while they play their instruments. Have writing materials accessible and encourage them to use their own notations to record their music or songs on paper, so that they can repeat it again at will or share it with others.
♦ Provide plenty of floor space so that the child can move, jig or dance to each other's music. Gather the group together, at the end of the session, to sing a favourite song while a band of children accompany it with instruments.
♦ Further develop the activity in subsequent sessions by adding a tape recorder for the children to use to record and listen to their own creations. You can also add songbooks to the display and encourage the children to use them to inspire their music.

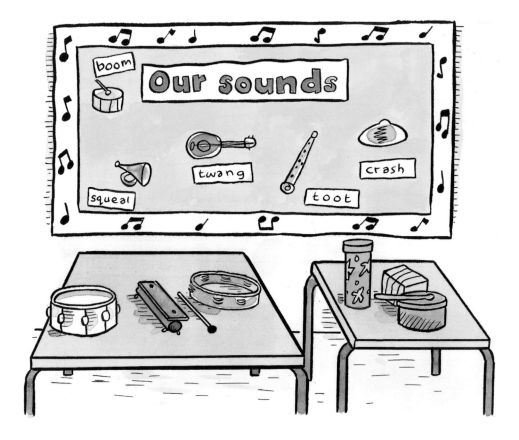

Perfect pizzas

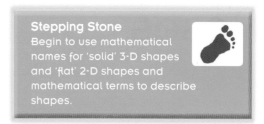

What you need
A selection of child-made 'pizzas' in different shapes and sizes (see the activity 'Pick a pizza' on page 59); frieze paper; table; play dough; separate containers of small yellow card triangles and rectangles, and small red, pink and green card circles; labels; marker pen.

Preparation
Back the wall with frieze paper and add a title, such as 'Perfect pizzas'.

What to do
Invite the children who made the pizzas to help you to display them attractively on the wall. Help them to make up names for their pizzas and write them on labels to go alongside them on the wall, for example, 'Peter's pepperoni', 'Millie's mini-pizza' and 'Phil's four seasons'.

Place the table in front of the display, but at a distance of between 1.5m to 2m from it, like a shop counter. Put the play dough and card shapes on the table and gather the group around.

Using the display
♦ Look at the wall display and talk about the pizzas using mathematical terms.
♦ Read the labels together and talk about who made the pizzas, how they made them and what they have called them.
♦ Explain that there is another way to make similar pizzas and show the children the play dough. Demonstrate how to break off a suitably sized piece, roll it into a ball and flatten it between your hands to make a thick or thin pizza base.
♦ Talk about the card shapes and what ingredients they represent as you create a pizza of your own. Explain to the children that they can change their pizzas very easily, by removing some of the topping and adding a different 'ingredient', and when they have finished, they can dismantle it completely and roll the dough back into a ball for someone else to use.
♦ As the children work, occasionally refer them to the display board to compare their creations with those on the wall. Discuss the shape and thickness of the base, for example, 'Can anyone make a base that is not round?'. Then ask the children to solve the following problem: two people wanting to share a pizza but liking different things.
♦ Add plastic knives, so that the children can practise dividing different shapes into different numbers of equal parts. At the end, ask volunteers to tidy up the table, wrap the dough and sort all the ingredients into the appropriate containers.

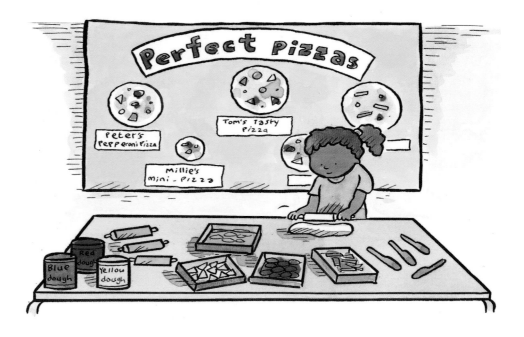

Noses

Stepping Stone
Display high levels of involvement in activities.

Early Learning Goal
Continue to be interested, excited and motivated to learn.

What you need
Frieze paper; book of noses made by the children (see the activity 'Our book of noses' on page 67); card or stiff paper in grey, brown and yellow; scissors; broad felt-tipped pens; large label; stapler or sticky tape; two tables; fabric; mirrors; selection of fake noses (home-made and/or commercially produced); recyclable materials, such as egg-boxes and small pots and containers; glue; shirring elastic or strong thread; awl (adult use).

Preparation
Cover the display board with frieze paper and write 'Noses' on a large label in the centre. Place the fake noses and mirrors on a table in front of it, but keep it covered with the fabric. Position the other table to one side to use as a craft table.

What to do
Look at the board together and read the word in the centre. Talk for a while about noses and look at the nose book created by the children.

Suggest that they make some animal masks with different sorts of noses: long elephant noses, tiny mouse noses, flat gorilla noses and so on. Help the children to create masks of their chosen animals using the coloured card and recyclable materials, and involve them in displaying them on the prepared wall.

Using the display
◆ Look at the masks and, again, spend some time talking about noses and what they are used for. Then uncover the fake noses and invite the children to try them on and look at themselves in the mirrors. Encourage each child to find a favourite nose and explain why they like it the most.
◆ Draw the children's attention to the craft table and recyclable materials, and invite them to make fake noses or masks of their own. Use the awl to punch holes for the children to thread shirring elastic or strong thread through, to hold the masks or noses in position.
◆ Encourage the children to talk to one another about what they are doing, asking for one another's opinions about what they look like or which nose suits them the most.
◆ At the end of the session, invite each child to select a nose or mask to wear while you recite together the rhyme 'My nose' on page 85.

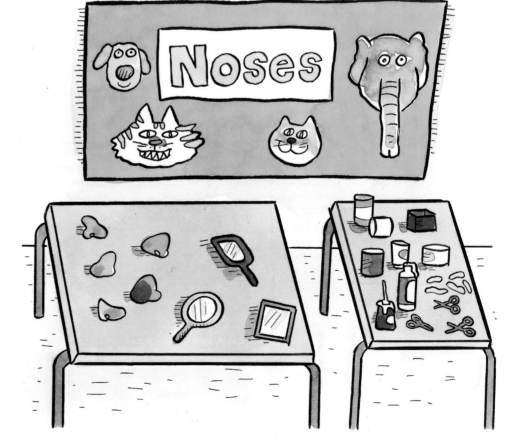

Rhymes

Wouldn't it be a funny world?

Wouldn't it be a funny world if things were changed around?
I'd listen with my eyes
and feel with my ears
and my nose would see the ground.
My hands would taste things if they liked – and maybe eat as well.
And that would leave my waggly tongue with nothing to do but smell!

But I don't think that seems quite right – I like it as it is.
With eyes to see
and ears to hear
and hands to stroke my Ted.
A nose to smell all sorts of scents and a tongue to taste fresh bread.

Barbara J Leach

My eyes

My eyes can wink *(close one eye)*
My eyes can blink *(close both eyes)*
My eyes can close to help me think. *(screw up eyes and look pensive)*

My eyes can stare *(stare)*
My eyes can glare *(look cross and glare)*
My eyes can close when I am scared. *(raise shoulders, screw up face and shut eyes tight)*

My eyes can weep *(brush away tears)*
My eyes can peep *(peep between fingers)*
My eyes can close to help me sleep. *(tip head to one side and gently close eyes)*

Barbara J Leach

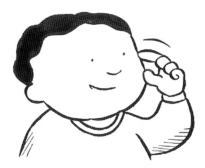

How does it feel?

How does it feel... (x2)
How does it feel... to... stroke a cat?
      It's soft and warm and snuggly, (x2)
      It's soft and warm and snuggly... and that is that.
How does it feel... (x2)
How does it feel... to... touch some ice?
      It's cold and wet and slippery, (x2)
      It's cold and wet and slippery... and that's not nice.
How does it feel... (x2)
How does it feel... to... hug a tree?
      It's hard and rather knobbly, (x2)
      It's hard and rather knobbly... don't you agree?
How does it feel... (x2)
How does it feel... to... touch some hair?
      It's soft and rather tickly, (x2)
      It's soft and rather tickly... ginger, dark or fair.

Barbara J Leach

Peace and quiet

Listen very carefully, be quiet as a mouse.
What can you hear **out**side your house?
Traffic rushing,
Water gushing,
Sirens shrieking,
People speaking,
Mowers humming,
Children running...
Help! It's too noisy – let's go indoors.

Listen very carefully, be quiet as a mouse.
What can you hear **in**side your house?
Telly blaring,
Kids not sharing,
Doorbell ringing,
Sister singing,
Baby crying,
Mummy sighing...
Oh no! It's too noisy. Where **can** I go for a bit of peace and quiet?

Barbara J Leach

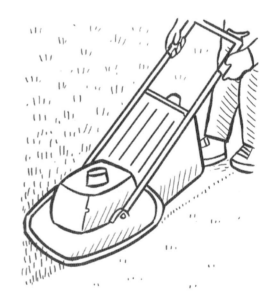

SCHOLASTIC Photocopiable

Foundation
Themes
Senses

A riddle

Can you think of something good to eat?
It isn't fruit and it isn't meat. *(pause a few seconds to think)*
It isn't a sandwich; it isn't a cake –
But you can put it inside the oven to bake. *(pause for thought again)*
It isn't a pancake; it isn't a tomato *(use the American pronunciation)*
You can chip it, you can mash it – you've guessed –

A POTATO!

Barbara J Leach

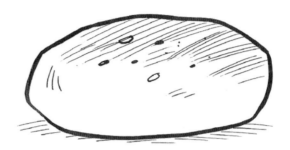

My nose

My nose is small and wriggly too.
It has some nostrils – I think there's two. *(point to nostrils)*
It can sniff, it can twitch, *(sniff and twitch your nose)*
It can tickle and itch, *(waggle and rub your nose)*
It sometimes makes... me... *(prepare for a sneeze)*
SNEEZE! *(cover your nose and sneeze)*
I like my nose, it's part of my face.
I really wouldn't want it in another place.
Would you? *(talk about what it would be
like to have your nose in another place, for example, on
top of your head or on your tummy)*

Barbara J Leach

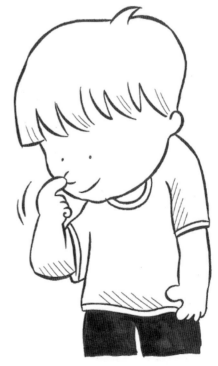

Songs

Things I can do

(Tune: 'In and Out the Dusky Bluebells')

I can see things with my eyes, (x3) *(point to eyes)*
I can see a... *(name and point at something you can see)*

I can hear things with my ears, (x3) *(cup ears)*
I can hear... *(cup hand behind ear and name something you can hear)*

I can smell things with my nostrils, (x3) *(gently tap nostrils)*
I can smell... *(name something and pinch nostrils or take a deep sniff depending on the aroma!)*

I can touch things with my fingers, (x3) *(wiggle fingers)*
I can touch... *(name something and make stroking action or quickly move hand away accordingly)*

I can taste things with my tongue, (x3) *(waggle tongue)*
I can taste... *(name something and rub tummy appreciatively or screw up face accordingly)*

Barbara J Leach

Can you?

(Tune: 'I Can Hear My Hands Go Clap, Clap, Clap')

Can you make your eyes go blink, blink, blink?
Can you make your eyes go wink, wink, wink?
Can you make your eyes look up and down?
Can you make your eyes go round and round?
Can you make your eyes to open wide?
Can you move your eyes from side to side?
Can you close your eyes up really tight?
Now go to sleep and say 'Good-night'.

Barbara J Leach

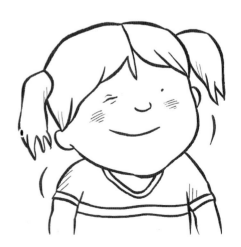

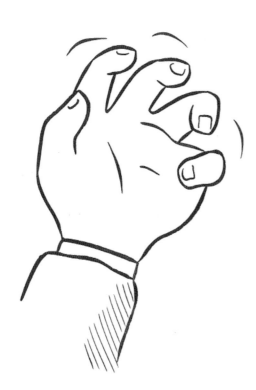

Touch

(Tune: 'Frère Jacques')

With your fingers. With your fingers,
You can touch. You can touch.
This is how it works now. This is how it works now.
Through your skin. Through your skin.

When you touch things. When you touch things.
With your skin. With your skin.
It sends along some messages. It sends along some
        messages.
To your brain. To your brain.

Your brain tells you. Your brain tells you.
What to feel. What to feel.
Hot or rough or prickly, cold or smooth or tickly.
You will know. You will know.

Barbara J Leach

Listen very carefully

(Tune: 'Polly Put the Kettle on')

Listen very carefully, *(put hand behind ear)*
Listen very carefully,
Listen very carefully,
What can you hear? *(adult meows)*
        I think it is a pussy cat, (x3)
        That wants some milk.

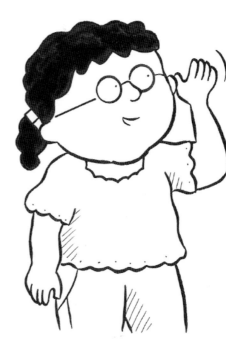

Listen very carefully, *(put hand behind ear)*
Listen very carefully,
Listen very carefully,
What can you hear? *(adult grunts)*
        I think it is a hungry pig, (x3)
        That wants some food.

Listen very carefully, *(put hand behind ear)*
Listen very carefully,
Listen very carefully,
What can you hear? *(adult trumpets and makes a trunk with their arm)*
        I think it is an elephant, (x3)
        That's big and strong.

(Continue adding verses at will, inviting the children to make the sounds.)

Barbara J Leach

Sugar is sweet

(Tune: 'Lavender's Blue')

Sugar is sweet dilly dilly,
Choc'late is too.
Here's some for me dilly dilly, *('eat' a piece of chocolate, wearing a suitable facial expression)*
And some for you. *(pretend to pass some chocolate to a friend)*

Lemons are sour dilly dilly,
Grapefruit is too.
Here's some for me dilly dilly, *('eat' grapefruit while screwing up your face)*
And some for you. *(pretend to pass some to a friend)*

Crisps taste of salt dilly dilly,
Chips, they do too.
Here's one for me dilly dilly, *('eat' one and lick salt off your lips)*
And one for you. *(pretend to pass one to a friend)*

(Make the song more fun by having samples of food to taste.)

Barbara J Leach

I can smell

(Tune: 'Three Blind Mice')

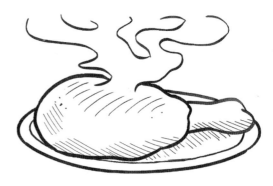

I can smell. *(sniff delicately)*
I can smell. *(sniff delicately)*
What can you smell?
What can you smell?
I can smell something that's not very sweet. *(wrinkle nose and look around)*
It might be the traffic fumes out in the street, *(point outside)*
Or maybe it's something that's stuck to my feet! *(look at soles of shoes)*
It sure does smell! *(hold nose and say, 'Phew!')*

I can smell. *(sniff delicately)*
I can smell. *(sniff delicately)*
What can you smell?
What can you smell?
I can smell something – I think it's a treat. *(look pleasantly surprised)*
It might be some chicken or other roast meat,
I am very hungry, I'd like some to eat. *(rub tummy and look hungry)*
Would you too? *(offer food to someone)*

(Variation: divide the group into two and sing alternate lines in turn.)

Barbara J Leach

Shape trails

Follow the shapes and write in the missing numbers.

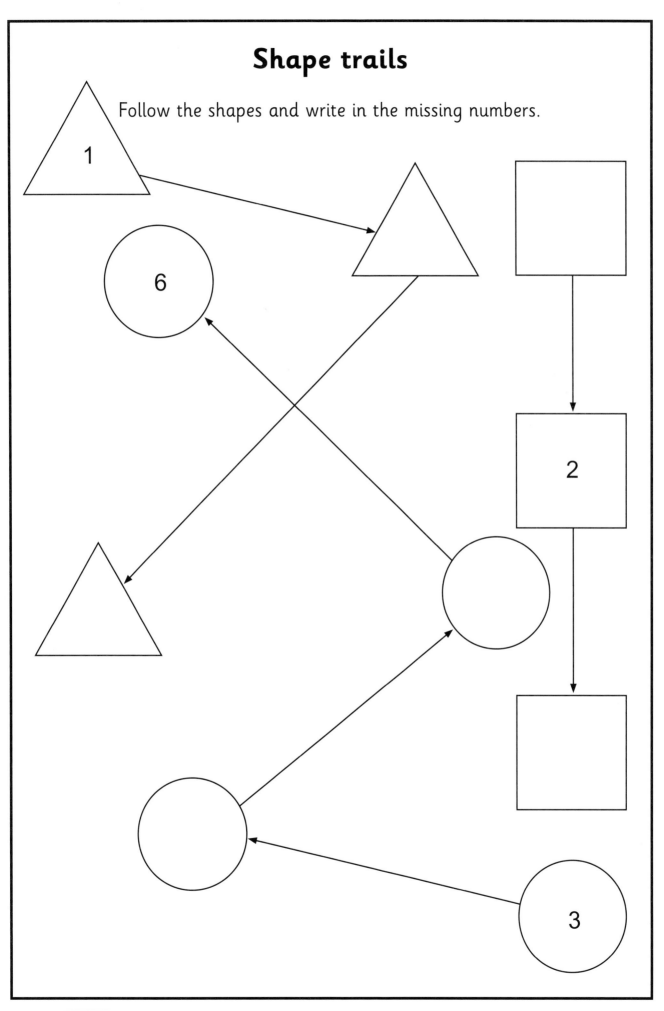

Eye chart

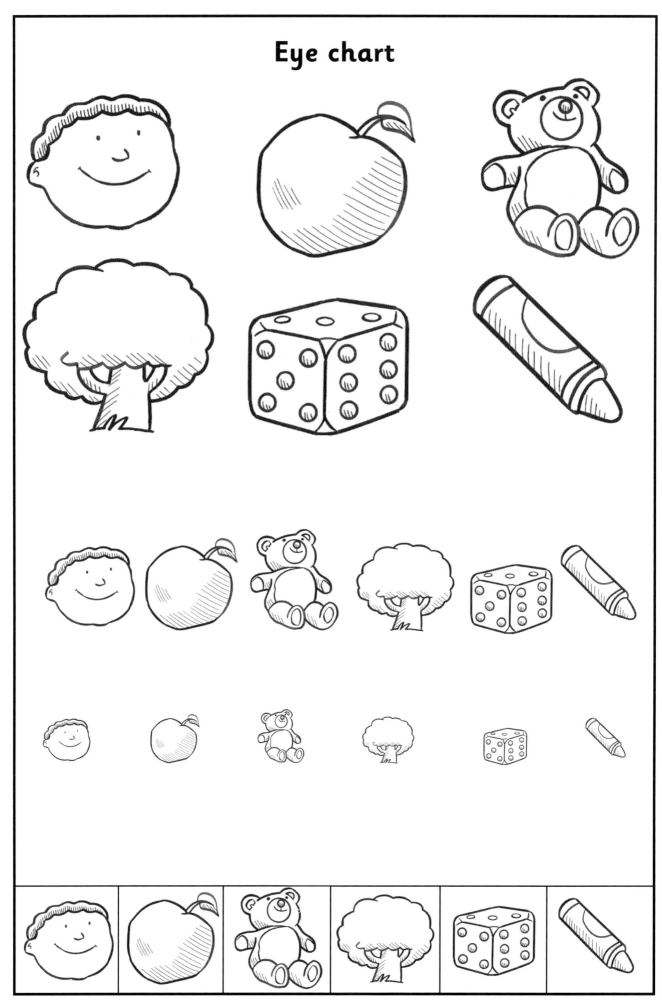

Foundation Themes

Senses

Roll and count

1	4	3	2
3	2	1	4

4	1	3	2
2	3	4	1

How far does it travel?

We measured how far the sound travelled from these instruments.

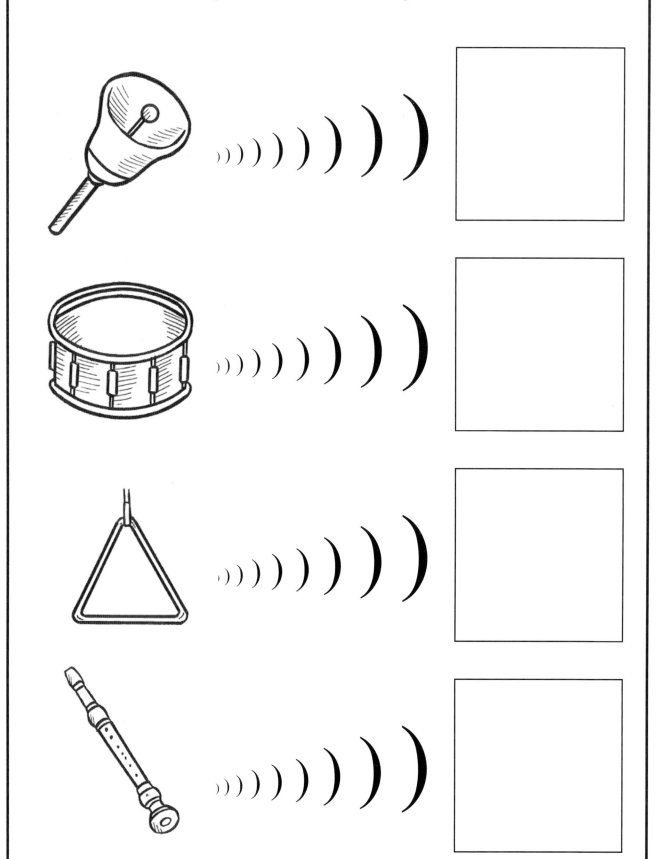

Match the fruit

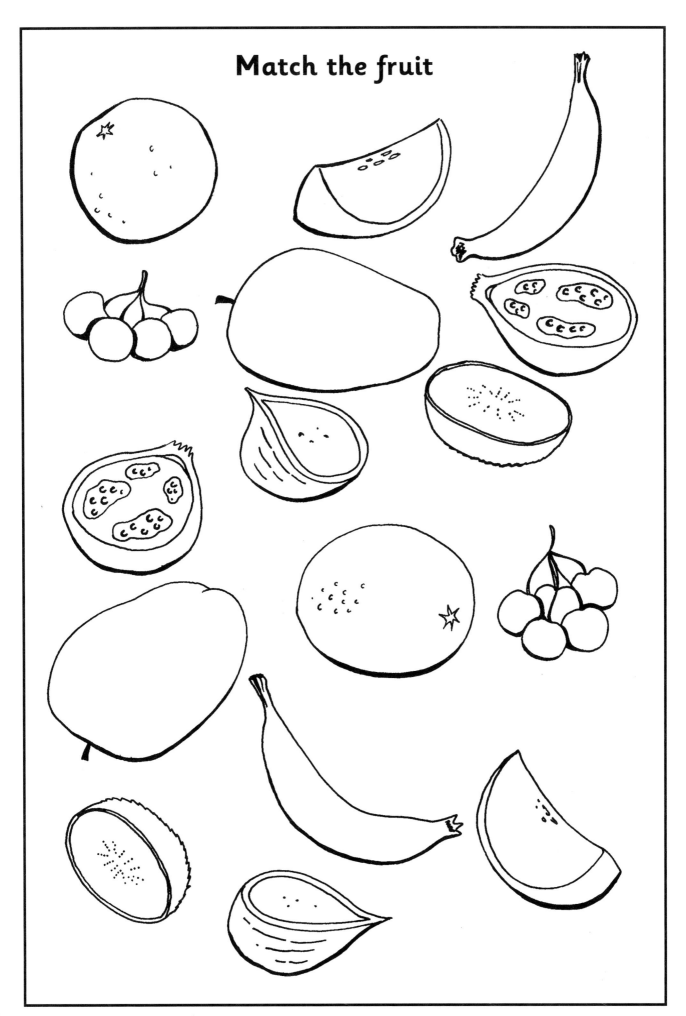

Food pairs

Find pairs of food that start with the same sound and talk about what they might taste like if eaten together. Colour them carefully.

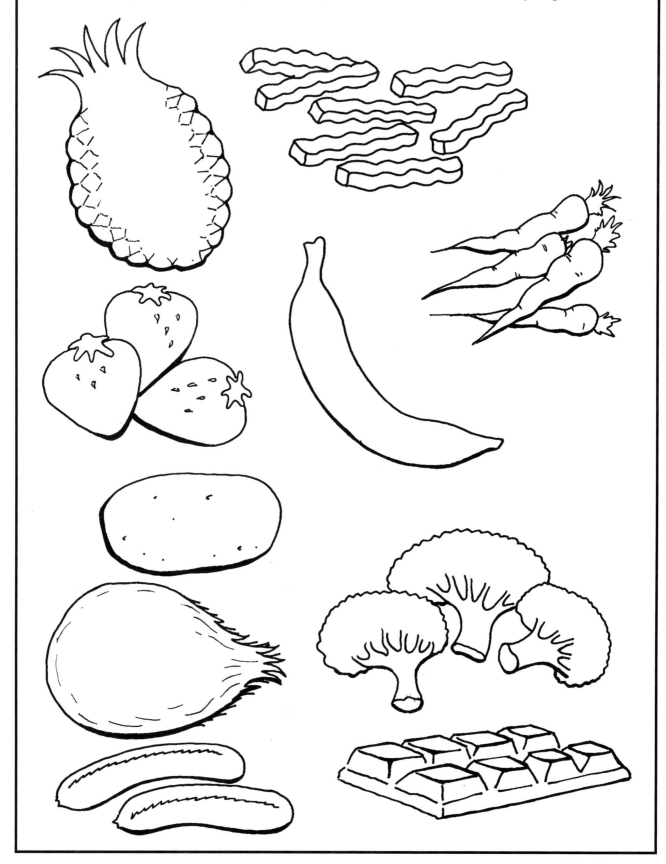

Sunflowers

Count the petals on each sunflower and write the number on the pot.

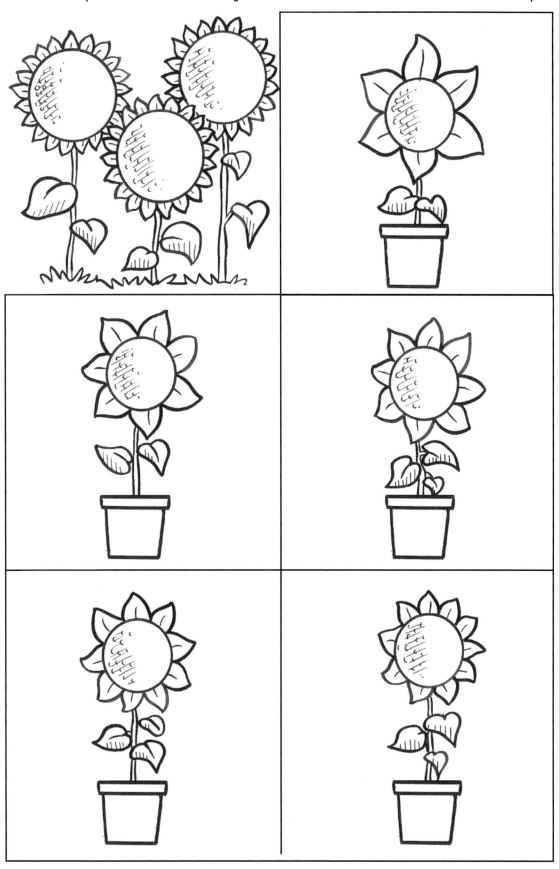

My garden

Add some flowers, plants, leaves and insects to complete your garden.

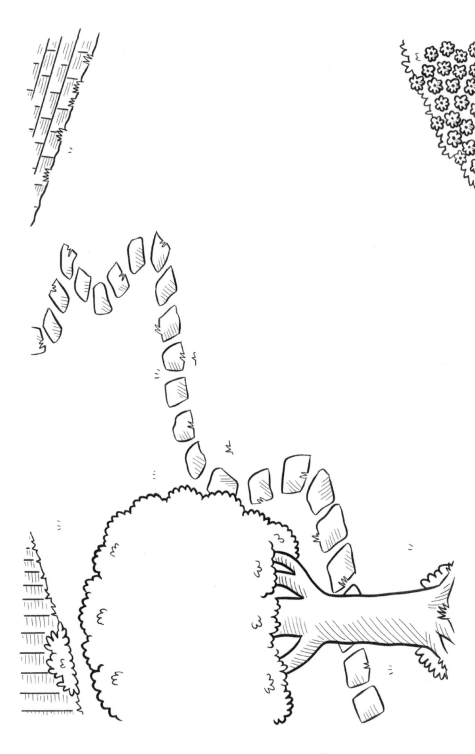